Acanthamoeba Keratitis

Xuguang Sun

Acanthamoeba Keratitis

Diagnosis and Treatment

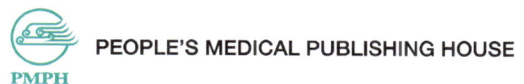 PEOPLE'S MEDICAL PUBLISHING HOUSE

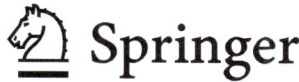 Springer

Xuguang Sun
Beijing Institute of Ophthalmology
Beijing Tongren Eye Center
Beijing Tongren Hospital
Capital Medical University
Beijing, China

Jointly published with People's Medical Publishing House

ISBN 978-981-10-5211-8   ISBN 978-981-10-5212-5   (eBook)
https://doi.org/10.1007/978-981-10-5212-5

The print edition is not for sale in China Mainland. Customers from China Mainland please order the print book from: People's Medical Publishing House.

Library of Congress Control Number: 2017964314

Printed on acid-free paper

This Springer imprint is published by Springer Nature
The registered company is Springer Nature Singapore Pte Ltd.
The registered company address is: 152 Beach Road, #21-01/04 Gateway East, Singapore 189721, Singapore

This book is dedicated to Professor Xiaolou Zhang (1914–1990), who set up the Department of Ocular Microbiology at the Beijing Institute of Ophthalmology in China.

Preface

As early as 1755, German scientist Rosel Von Rosenhof made the first observation of a *free-living amoeba* in detail. However, no attention was paid to explore the relationship between human diseases and this organism in the following two hundred years. In 1958, Professor Culbertson et al. found during a vaccine safety test that free-living amoebae could result in the infection of the central nervous system of animals. Thus, he predicted that free-living amoebae would become one of the pathogens of human diseases, which was confirmed by Australian scientist Fowler M and colleagues in 1965, who reported the case of human infection caused by free-living amoebae for the first time in the world.

In 1974, Naginton J et al. reported the first case of *Acanthamoeba* keratitis in the world. In China, Professor Xiuying Jin and her colleagues from the Beijing Institute of Ophthalmology published a case report of *Acanthamoeba* keratitis in Ophthalmology in China in 1992, which was considered the first article about *Acanthamoeba* keratitis published by Chinese scientists. In the subsequent 20 years, ophthalmologists and researchers in the Department of Ocular Microbiology at the Beijing Institute of Ophthalmology have been involved in related basic and clinical research on *Acanthamoeba* keratitis. More than 300 cases of this disease on the basis of etiological diagnosis were collected. In addition, over 170 strains of *Acanthamoeba* spp. were stored in the laboratory. Moreover, a series of studies were carried out that mainly focused on the biological characteristics of *Acanthamoeba*, pathological mechanisms, clinical and laboratory diagnosis, as well as anti-amoebic drugs and surgical treatments.

The *Acanthamoeba* pathogen is widely distributed in nature. But as a type of rare ocular infection, *Acanthamoeba* accounts only for about 5% of the pathogens that may lead to *suppurative corneal infection* according to the data from the Beijing Institute of Ophthalmology. However, *Acanthamoeba* keratitis is generally considered as a type of *sight-threatening* keratitis that is difficult to treat. At the early stages, *Acanthamoeba* keratitis usually shows atypical clinical manifestations, which are often misdiagnosed as viral or bacterial keratitis. Moreover, there are no approved topical anti-amoebic drugs available to date. The number of patients might further increase due to the increasing populations using corneal contact lens in the world. It is necessary for ophthalmological practitioners to have a comprehensive understanding of this infection from several perspectives including characteristics of pathogen, risk factors, clinical manifestations, diagnosis, and treatment.

This book provides brief and concise descriptions of the basic and clinical knowledge about *Acanthamoeba* keratitis with abundant figure illustrations and typical cases to ophthalmological practitioners and researchers.

Beijing, China   Xuguang Sun
Beijing, China   Zhiqun Wang
2017

Acknowledgments

On the occasion of publishing this book, we would like to express our sincere gratitude to Professors Xiuying Jin and Wenhua Zhang from the Department of Ocular Microbiology at the Beijing Institute of Ophthalmology and the Beijing Tongren Ophthalmology Center. We are grateful for the important preliminary work that they along with their colleagues have done in the diagnosis and treatment of *Acanthamoeba* keratitis, which paved the way to further in-depth and continuous research on this disease in China.

We also greatly appreciate the invaluable support given by colleagues of the corneal group in the Beijing Tongren Ophthalmology Center in providing surgical therapy of *Acanthamoeba* keratitis. In addition, we express our sincere thanks to Professor Bin Li and his colleagues from the pathology laboratory of the Beijing Institute of Ophthalmology for their ardent assistance in corneal pathological diagnosis and research on *Acanthamoeba*.

Furthermore, we express our heartfelt gratitude to the doctors and graduate students of the Beijing Institute of Ophthalmology, including Aixue Zhang, Rui Gao, Xiaoyu Zhang, Jinghao Qu, and Li Li, who put in great efforts in proofreading and verifying statistics of the data in this book.

Finally we also express our thanks to all the *Acanthamoeba* keratitis patients who have gone through our treatments for their understanding of and cooperation with our clinical studies.

Contributors: Wei Chen, Shijing Deng, Min Gao, Chao Jiang , Ran Li, Qingfeng Liang, Chang Liu, ShiyunLuo, Chen Zhang, Xiaoyan Zhang, Yan Zhang, Yang Zhang

Contents

About the Authors

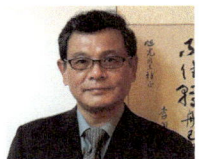 **Xuguang Sun** is chair and professor in the Department of Ocular Microbiology at Beijing Institute of Ophthalmology and also works at the Beijing Tongren Ophthalmology Center. He has been engaged in clinical and research work on the corneal diseases and infectious ocular diseases since 1986.

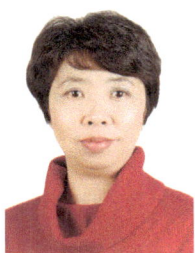 **Zhiqun Wang** is associate chief technician in the Department of Ocular Microbiology at Beijing Institute of Ophthalmology and also works at the Beijing Tongren Ophthalmology Center. She has been working at the clinical laboratory for Ocular Microbiological research work since 1989.

In 1974, the first case of *Acanthamoeba keratitis* was reported in scientific literature [1]. Although group occurrences of this disease have been reported from certain regions, *Acanthamoeba* keratitis is still generally considered as a type of rare disease compared to bacterial and fungal keratitis, as listed in Table 1.1.

After the 1980s, the clinical cognition and laboratory diagnosis level of this disease was gradually improved. In addition, the population of corneal contact lens wearers rapidly increased. As a consequence, the diagnosed cases of *Acanthamoeba* keratitis increased significantly. It has been observed that the incidence of *Acanthamoeba* keratitis differed among the countries or different regions of the country, which is mainly associated with the population of corneal contact lens wearers, risk factors, climate, sanitation state of tap water, the distribution and virulence of *Acanthamoeba* strains, etc. [2].

1.1   Incidence in Developed Countries and Regions

The statistical report in 1989 showed that the estimated incidence of *Acanthamoeba* keratitis was 1.36 per million in the United States of America [3]. The annual incidence of this disease in England and Wales was 1.26 (1997–1998) and 1.13 (1998–1999) per

Table 1.1 Distribution of pathogens in suppurative keratitis from 1989 to 2006 in Beijing Institute of Ophthalmology

Pathogen	No. examined samples	No. culture positive	Culture positive rate %	Percent (%)[a]
Bacteria	5995	1161	19.37	40.09
Fungus	4735	1602	33.83	55.32
Acanthamoeba	572	133	23.25	4.59
Total	11,302	2896		100.00

[a]Percent (%): No. culture positive/Total no. culture positive × 100%

© Springer Nature Singapore Pte Ltd.
& People's Medical Publishing House, PR of China 2018
X. Sun, *Acanthamoeba Keratitis*, https://doi.org/10.1007/978-981-10-5212-5_1

million adults, respectively. Among the population of corneal contact lens wearers, the incidence increased dramatically to 31 and 27 per million in England and Wales, respectively, 88% of which were hydrogel contact lens wearers [4, 5]. The annual incidence of *Acanthamoeba* keratitis was one per 40,000 people in New Zealand as reported in 1995 [6] and was 33 per million in Hong Kong (1997–1998) [7].

In developed countries and regions, corneal contact lens wear is the first *risk factor* for *Acanthamoeba* keratitis. With the popularization of knowledge concerning contact lenses and popular application of effective lens care solution, gradual decrease was observed in the number of cases of this disease since 1995 [8].

1.2   Incidence in Developing Countries and Regions

According to a report from South India, the incidence of *Acanthamoeba* keratitis among elderly patients was 1.4% with no relation to corneal contact lens wear. Across the whole Indian subcontinent, only 4.5% of *Acanthamoeba* keratitis patients showed the correspondence between the disease and the wear of contact lens [9, 10].

Xiuying Jin et al. from Beijing Institute of Ophthalmology reported a case of *Acanthamoeba* keratitis in 1992, which was the first case of this disease in Mainland of China. By the end of 2008, approximately 300 cases were reported in Chinese medical journals [11]. From 1991 to 2015, 304 cases of *Acanthamoeba* keratitis on the basis of etiological diagnosis were collected by Beijing Institute of Ophthalmology, as reported in Table 1.2. Among these, 53.8% of the cases were related with ocular traumas and 29.1% with corneal contact lens wear [12]. Therefore, different from that in developed countries, the first *risk factor* of the disease in developing countries was ocular traumas, especially vegetal traumas, or the splash of contaminated water, followed by corneal contact lens wear. Up to now, there is no published epidemiological data about the incidence of *Acanthamoeba* keratitis in Mainland of China.

Table 1.2 304 cases of *Acanthamoeba* keratitis diagnosed by Beijing Institute of Ophthalmology from 1991 to 2015

Years	No. cases	Percent (%)
1991–1995	13	4.3
1996–2000	34	11.2
2001–2005	80	26.3
2006–2010	80	26.3
2011–2015	97	31.9
Total	304	100.0

References

1. Naginton J, Watson PG, Playfair TJ, et al. Amoebic infection of the eye. Lancet. 1974;2(7896):1537–40.
2. Ibrahim YW, Boase DL, Cree IA. Factors affecting the epidemiology of Acanthamoeba keratitis. Ophthalmic Epidemiol. 2007;14(2):53–60.
3. Poggio EC, Glynn RJ, Schein OD, et al. The incidence of ulcerative keratitis among users of daily-wear and extended-wear soft contact lenses. N Engl J Med. 1989;321(12):779–83.
4. Seal DV. Acanthamoeba keratitis update-incidence, molecular epidemiology and new drugs for treatment. Eye. 2003;17(8):893–905.
5. Radford CF, Minassian DC, Dart JK. Acanthamoeba keratitis in England and Wales: incidence, outcome, and risk factors. Br J Ophthalmol. 2002;86(5):536–42.
6. Murdoch D, Gray TB, Cursons R, et al. Acanthamoeba keratitis in New Zealand, including two cases with in vivo resistance to polyhexamethylene biguanide. Aust N Z J Ophthalmol. 1998;26(3):231–6.
7. Lam DS, Houang E, Fan DS, et al. Incidence and risk factors for microbial keratitis in Hong Kong: comparison with Europe and North America. Eye (Lond.). 2002;16(5):608–18.
8. Morlet N, Duguid G, Radford C, et al. Incidence of Acanthamoeba keratitis associated with contact lens wear. Lancet. 1997;350(9075):414.
9. Sharma S, Gopalakrishnan S, Aasuri MK, et al. Trends in contact lens-associated microbial keratitis in Southern India. Ophthalmology. 2003;110(1):138–43.
10. Kunimoto DY, Sharma S, Garg P, et al. Corneal ulceration in the elderly in Hyderabad, South India. Br J Ophthalmol. 2000;84(1):54–9.
11. Gao M, Sun XG. Pathogenic free-living amoebic keratitis in China. [Article in Chinese]. Zhonghua Yan Ke Za Zhi. 2006;42(1):64–7.
12. Li L, Liang Y, Zhang C, et al. Etiological study suppurative keratitis. Recent Adv Ophthalmol. 2008;28(10):749–52.

Free-living amoeba refers to a group of amoebic protozoa that are able to survive and reproduce with their own biological metabolism system instead of living within the host. The majority species of free-living amoeba existing in the environment does not induce the human infections, while a few species may survive and reproduce within insects, animals, and human beings under different kinds of conditions. They are called as facultative parasites. Subsequently, these species of free-living amoeba also termed as pathogenic free-living amoeba or an opportunistic pathogen medically, which may cause certain diseases in animals and humans [1].

2.1 Biological Characteristics of Free-Living Amoeba

According to taxonomy, amoeba is a type of unicellular protozoa with a simple biological structure, belonging to protozoan phylum, Lobosa class, and Amoebida order. There are mainly two medicine-related categories of amoebas, including *parasitic amoeba* and free-living amoeba.

Free-living amoeba is widely distributed in diverse natural environments as well as man-made environments. Free-living amoeba has been isolated from various natural water sources (such as lakes, rivers, seas, etc.), soil, dust, dirt, decayed plants, and suspended particles in the air. Besides, free-living amoeba also has been isolated from the bodies of insects, fishes, amphibians, reptiles, and other healthy and dead animals. In addition to the natural environments, free-living amoeba has been isolated from distilled water bottles, swimming pools, sewage pipes, tap water system, air conditioning units, and so on. Moreover, it has been discovered even from dental clinics, hospitals, dialysis units, and corneal contact lenses and their cases [2, 3]. This wide distribution of free-living amoeba suggested that people commonly encounter this organism in their routine lives.

© Springer Nature Singapore Pte Ltd.
& People's Medical Publishing House, PR of China 2018
X. Sun, *Acanthamoeba Keratitis*, https://doi.org/10.1007/978-981-10-5212-5_2

Pathogenic free-living amoeba related with ocular infections mainly includes *Acanthamoeba* spp. of *Acanthamoebida* family and *Naegleria* spp. of *Dimastiamoebidiae. Acanthamoeba* spp. is the most common pathogen for ocular infection, but a very few cases of corneal infection caused by *Naegleria* spp. were reported previously [4].

2.2   *Acanthamoeba* spp.

Acanthamoeba is the most common amoebic protozoan that induces ocular infection and usually exists in polluted soil or water sources. There are two forms of *Acanthamoeba* in its *life cycle*, i.e., an active *trophozoite* and a dormant *cyst*, which can transform each other under a given condition, as shown in Fig. 2.1.

2.2.1   Trophozoite

Trophozoite is the active form of *Acanthamoeba* protozoa, and trophozoite can reproduce by binary fission in optimal growth conditions and produce human infections under a given condition. Under light microscope, trophozoite is often round or oval in shape with a diameter of 15–45 μm (average 20 μm). The trophozoite often exhibits active movements with continuous changes in its shape. Thus, various shapes of trophozoite can be observed under a light microscope.

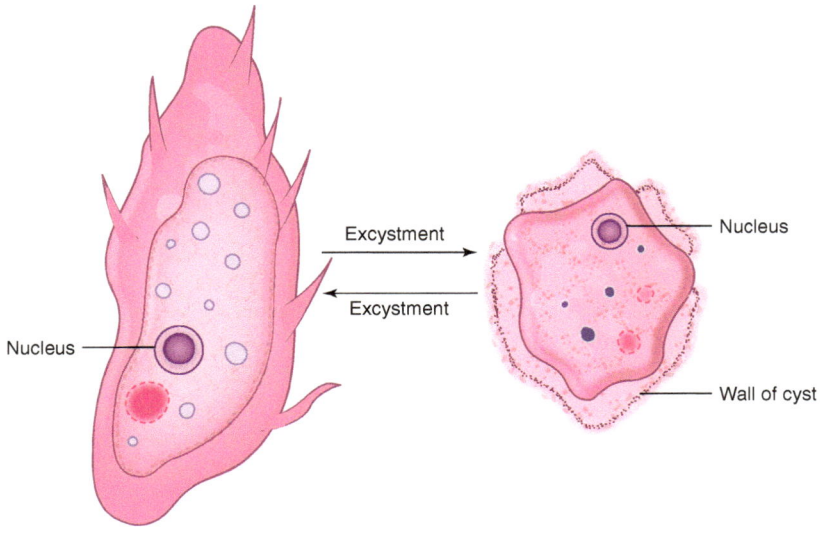

Fig. 2.1 There are two forms of *Acanthamoeba* in its life cycle, i.e., an active trophozoite and a dormant cyst, which can transform each other under a given condition

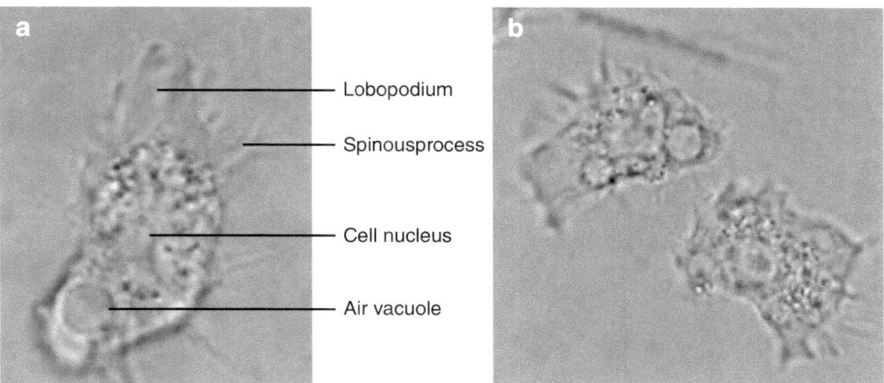

Fig. 2.2 (**a, b**) Trophozoites of *Acanthamoeba* with cell nucleus, spinous process, and air vacuole (×1000)

Trophozoite is covered by a thin cell membrane, and the *cytoplasm* of trophozoite contains various components, including much *lipid droplet*, *food vacuole*, and *liquid vacuole*. Abundant *mitochondria* can be observed clearly in the cytoplasm of trophozoite. The cell *nucleus* with a diameter of 6 μm is usually located in the center of trophozoite cell, and its nuclear chromatin is hypochromatic. A round and compact *nucleolus* with a diameter of 2.4 μm can be detected in the middle of the cell nucleus and is surrounded by transparent banding area. Nucleolus and its transparent banding area comprise the characteristic cellular structures for *Acanthamoeba* [5], which are also the important structural marker in the diagnosis of clinical microbial morphology (Fig. 2.2).

When the growth conditions are optimal, i.e., abundant food supply and suitable temperatures, the movement and metabolism of trophozoite will become very active. There are many spiculate protuberances stretching from the surface of the cell membrane, which are called *spinous processes*. Spinous process is one of the important cellular structures that distinguish *Acanthamoeba* spp. from *Naegleria* spp. Normally, a *fan-shaped pseudopodium* (also called as *lobopodium*) is formed on the side of cell along which the trophozoite moves. Under light microscope, the lobopodium is transparent without granular materials, as shown in Fig. 2.2.

Under a *transmission electron microscope*, the cell membrane of trophozoite can be divided into three sub-layers. In the cytoplasm, freely distributed *ribosomes*, *tubular structures*, aggregated *fibrils*, varying amounts of *Golgi apparatus*, *smooth* and *rough endoplasmic reticulum*, *phagocytic vacuole*, and *liquid vacuole* or *contractile vacuole* can be observed. In addition, an abundant mitochondria, lipid droplets, *lysosomes*, and *glycogen granules* are also found in the cytoplasm. On some circumstances, other kinds of microorganisms such as symbiotic bacteria may be detected in the cytoplasm [2]. Using the scanning electron microscope, trophozoite is round, oval, or irregular in shape with a diameter of around 15–45 μm. Its surface is rough with a large number of cone-shaped and *spinous processes* (Fig. 2.3).

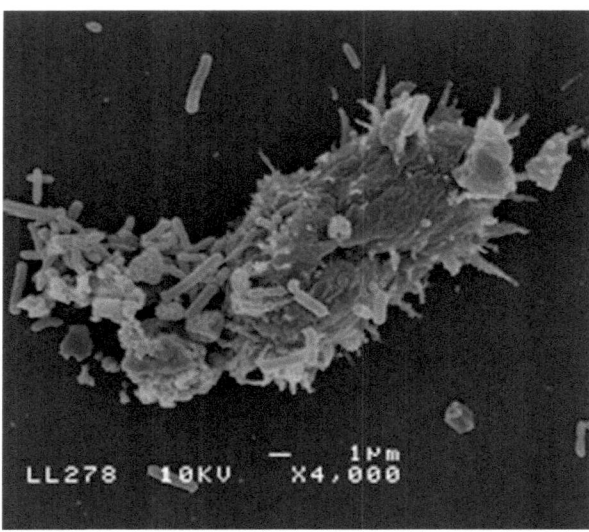

Fig. 2.3 Trophozoite is round, oval, or irregular in shape with many cone and spiculate processes on its surface (×4000)

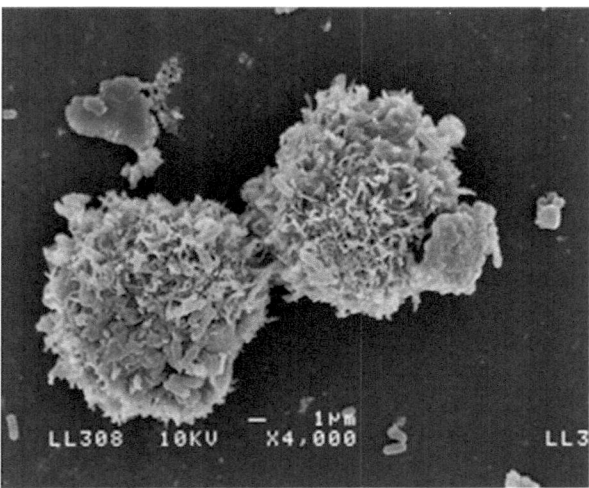

Fig. 2.4 Trophozoite reproduces by binary fission (×4000). Two daughter trophozoites are formed

Trophozoite reproduces by binary fission (as illustrated in Fig. 2.4) with an average *fissiparity cycle* time of about 10 h (ranging from 6 to 24 h). During the early prophase of binary fission, the cell nucleolus firstly ruptures itself and gradually disappears. Subsequently, the metaphase of binary fission starts in which chromatin forms a banding shape in the equatorial region and then is divided into two parts. Next, during the interphase, the centrosome in the shape of dense long column

Fig. 2.5 Binary fission state of *Acanthamoeba* trophozoite (by white arrow ×3000)

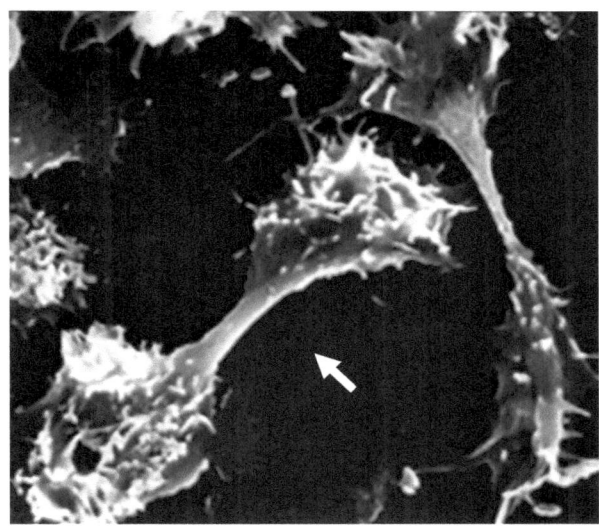

appears in the cytoplasm adjacent to the cell nucleus and adheres to tubular structures. The following phase of binary fission is the anaphase where chromatin in the form of dense and fine fibers immigrates and arrives at two poles of the cell. During the last phase (i.e., telophase), cell nuclear membrane reemerges, and this membrane surrounds two newly formed cell nuclei and then two cell nuclei separated along with the completion of cell division [3, 6], as demonstrated in Fig. 2.5. Finally two *daughter trophozoites* are formed.

Active *Acanthamoeba* can move freely and slowly in the direction of lobopodium, and its average *mobile velocity* in aqueous medium is estimated as 50 μm/min. Trophozoite generally feeds on bacteria, fungi, and other protozoa or marine algae for their survival. There are mainly two feeding methods: (1) *food cup sucking* and (2) phagocytizing liquid through *pinocytosis* (Fig. 2.6).

2.2.2 Cyst

In unfavorable conditions, i.e., desiccation and nutrient and oxygen deficiency, *Acanthamoeba* trophozoite can transform into a cyst gradually that is the relative dominant state of *Acanthamoeba* with very low metabolism rate, but it has powerful resistance to the natural environment as well as man-made environment. At the early phase of transforming, trophozoite gradually becomes smaller in size and more spherical. At the same time, trophozoite's mobility decreases and finally stops moving. Along with the dehydration of the cytoplasm, trophozoite begins to secrete and form a dense double-wall structure. Through prophase or immature period, i.e., *pre-cyst* or immature cyst (Fig. 2.7), trophozoite transformed into a mature cyst finally, and the duration of complete transformation from trophozoite to mature cyst generally needs several days.

Fig. 2.6 Huge
"pinocytotic vesicles" of
Acanthamoeba trophozoite
(shown by white arrow
×3000)

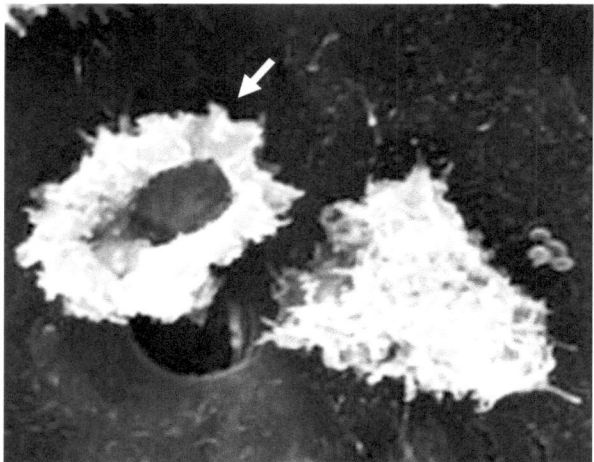

Fig. 2.7 Pre-cyst.
Acanthamoeba trophozoite
loses its pseudopodium
and spinous process and
becomes spherical in shape
(×1000)

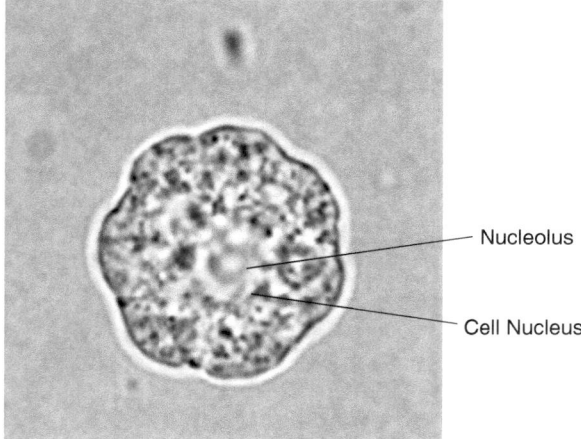

Nucleolus

Cell Nucleus

Cyst is generally round or oval in shape with a diameter of 10–25 μm. The mature cyst has a dense double wall, a wrinkled outer wall, and a smooth inner wall, and the latter has various shapes, such as polygon, circle, star, or triangle (Fig. 2.8a–e). The cytoplasm of a cyst contains a lot of dense granules comprised of abundant food particles, lipid droplets, glycogen, mitochondria, etc. The nucleus realm is not obvious, but porphyritic nucleolus can be observed clearly. The outer and inner walls normally are separated by a transparent band space. At some locations, the inner and outer walls of the cyst form opercula in the center of the *ostioles*, where excysting trophozoites will exit from. Depending on different strains of *Acanthamoeba*, the structure, amount, and distribution of the ostioles on the surface of double-walled cysts vary. The ostiole acts as the channel by which the cysts could monitor the

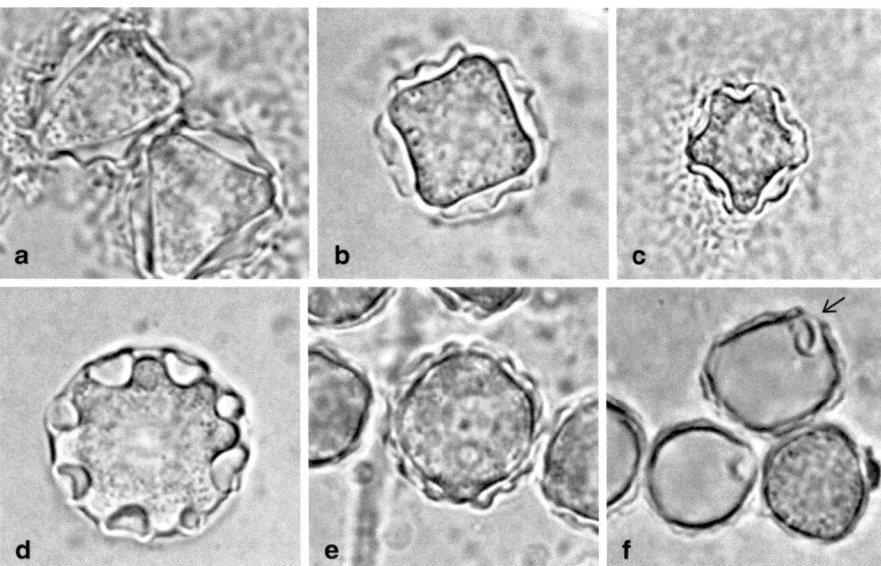

Fig. 2.8 (a–e) Cysts with dense double wall in various shapes (outer wall and inner wall). (f) Trophozoites excysts through the ostiole, with an empty double-wall shell without any contents in cyst (black arrow) (×1000)

external environment changes. Cysts begin to transform to trophozoite gradually under favorable conditions; the immature trophozoites emerge from cyst through the ostiole, leaving an empty double-wall shell without any contents in it (Fig. 2.8f). During the culture of *Acanthamoeba* in laboratory conditions, it takes from 10 to 24 h to finish the process of transformation from cyst to trophozoite. At present, initiation factors and mechanism of such transformation remain unclear.

Under the *transmission electron microscope*, typical double-wall structures of cyst can be observed. The outer wall is filled with fibrous wrinkled matrix material in distinct parallel structure. By contrast, the inner wall is a smooth polyhedron and composed of fine fibrils. These two layers of walls are separated by a structureless transparent band space (Fig. 2.9a). The ostioles formed by the fusion of the inner and outer walls usually arrange in the equatorial plane of the cyst. More specifically, the ostioles of pathogenic *Acanthamoeba* cysts show the microcrater-like type (Fig. 2.9b).

Under *scanning electron microscope*, the cyst is round with a diameter of around 10–25 μm. The surface of the cyst appears plicate, wavy, or wrinkled. Several slightly concave annular *spinous foramens* (the ostioles) can be observed on the capsule wall within certain intervals. The spinous foramens (the ostioles) are the pathway of *Acanthamoeba* immature trophozoites during *excystation* (Fig. 2.10). When the cover of spinosum foramen dissolves, *Acanthamoeba* immature trophozoite emerges from cyst through this pore and transforms into mature trophozoite (Fig. 2.11). After excystation, the empty shell of the cyst is left behind (Fig. 2.12).

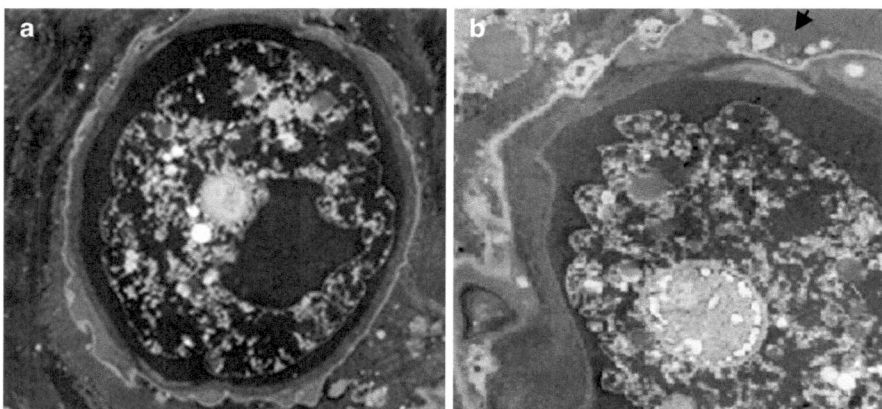

Fig. 2.9 (**a**) Cyst with the typical double-wall structure (×4000). (**b**) The microcrater-like ostiole of the cyst (black arrow) (×4000)

Fig. 2.10 The surface of the cyst appears plicate or wavy with the ostiole of the cyst (black arrow) (×5500)

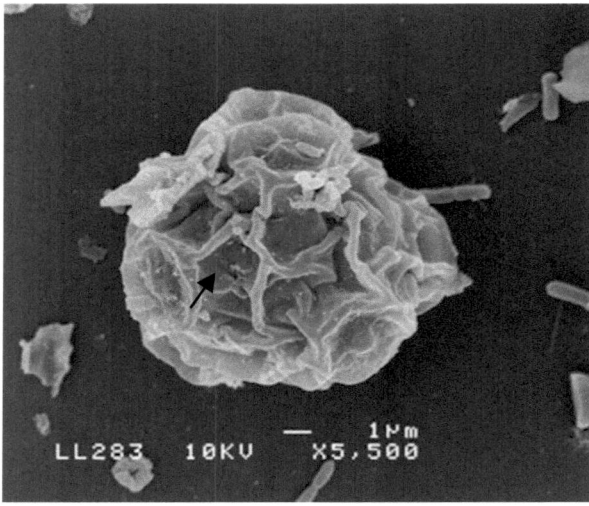

The *metabolic rate* of *Acanthamoeba* is rather low during its cystic period, which is almost in "hibernation" state. A cyst can withstand various physical and chemical factors in the environment, i.e., cold, heat, desiccation, a variety of disinfectants containing chlorine, and antibacterial drugs generally used. It has been shown that *Acanthamoeba* cyst can still survive in conditions with pH 3.9–pH 9.75 and temperature from −20 °C to 42 °C [7]. The cysts of some pathogenic *Acanthamoeba* strains, such as *A. castellanii*, can tolerate the temperature of 65 °C for 5 min or remain alive after being frozen and dissolved repeatedly for five times. In addition, it is able to resist the exposure of 250 K rad gamma ray radiation and the ultraviolet-B radiation of 800 mJ/mm^2. In the natural environment, cysts generally can remain viable for several years while maintaining their pathogenicity. In very special cases

Fig. 2.11 Excystation of *Acanthamoeba*. The empty shell of the cyst is left behind (white arrow), and immature trophozoite emerges from the ostiole (red arrow) (×4000)

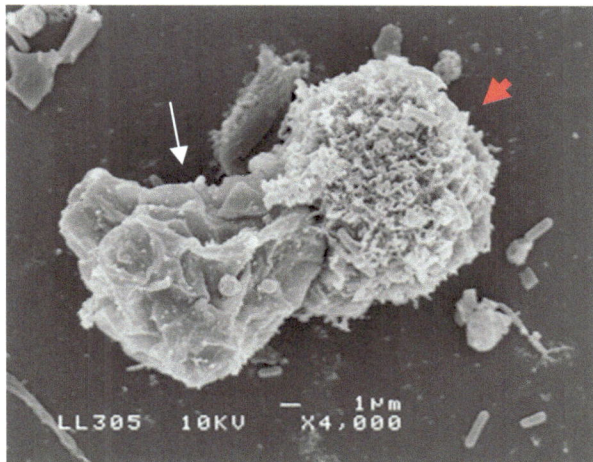

Fig. 2.12 Round hole and the cover of foramen are observed on the empty shell of the cyst after excystation, as indicated by the white arrow (×5000)

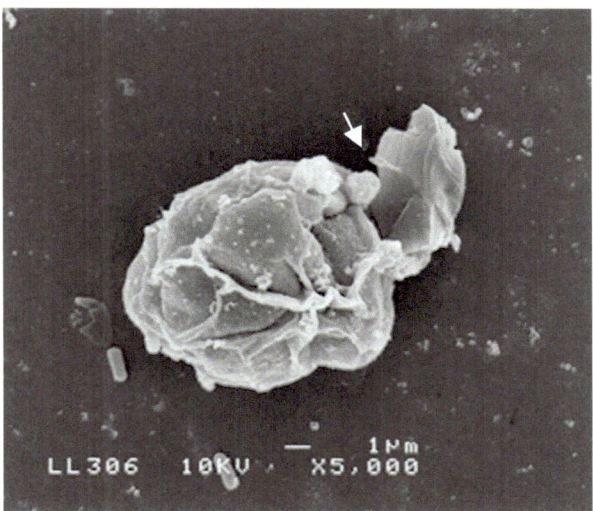

of *Acanthamoeba* keratitis, it has been reported that cysts can remain in the corneal tissues for up to 3 years [8].

2.2.3 Classification of *Acanthamoeba*

A total of 25 types of *Acanthamoeba* have been detected so far, at least 10 types of which may induce human keratitis, including *A. polyphaga, A. castellanii, A. culbertsoni, A. hatchetti, A. rhysodes, A. lugdunensis, A. quina, A. griffini, A. astronyxis, and A. triangularis.* In particular, *A. castellanii* and *A. polyphaga* and *A. culbertsoni* show the strongest pathogenic potential, which is assumed to be related with their adhesion ability to the corneal tissues, reproduction speed, and specific enzymatic activity [1].

- *Morphology Classification*: The shape of *Acanthamoeba* trophozoites displays a large variety because of their continuous movement, thus making it difficult to be considered as a basis for classification. However, morphological structures of *Acanthamoeba* cysts are relatively stable that differ by certain degrees among different groups of cysts. Therefore, *Acanthamoeba* is conventionally classified based on the morphological characteristics of the cyst forms. In 1967, Page categorized *Acanthamoeba* as an independent genus [8]. After a decade, *Pussard and Pons* classified *Acanthamoeba* genus (18 species in the time) into three groups according to morphology of the cyst forms in 1977. Subsequently, this classification scheme gained acceptance (Table 2.1) [1].

  Group I: The sizes of cysts are relatively larger of which the average diameter is 18 μm or more than 18 μm. There is a broader gap between the outer and inner walls. The outer wall is relatively smooth or wrinkled, whereas the inner wall shows a star-like shape (Fig. 2.13). There are four species in this group including *A. astronyxis*, *A. comandoni*, *A. echinulata*, and *A. tubiashi*.

  Group II: Eleven species were placed in this group which are widely distributed and commonly isolated in the natural and man-made environments. Usually the average diameter of cysts is less than 18 μm. The outer wall is usually wavy or mammilla, and the inner wall often forms different shapes including star-like, polygon or triangle, and round or oval. The distance between the outer wall and inner wall varies (Fig. 2.14).

Table 2.1 Classification of *Acanthamoeba* based on morphology

Morphology group	Name of types
Group I	A. astronyxis
	A. comandoni
	A. echinulata
	A. tubiashi
Group II	A. castellanii
	A. mauritaniensis
	A. polyphaga
	A. lugdunensis
	A. quina
	A. rhysodes
	A. divionensis
	A. paradivionensis
	A. griffini
	A. triangularis
	A. hatchetti
Group III	A. palestinensis
	A. culbertsoni
	A. lenticulata
	A. pustulosa
	A. royreba

Fig. 2.13 Group I: the
size of cysts in this group
is relatively larger with the
wrinkled outer wall
(×1000)

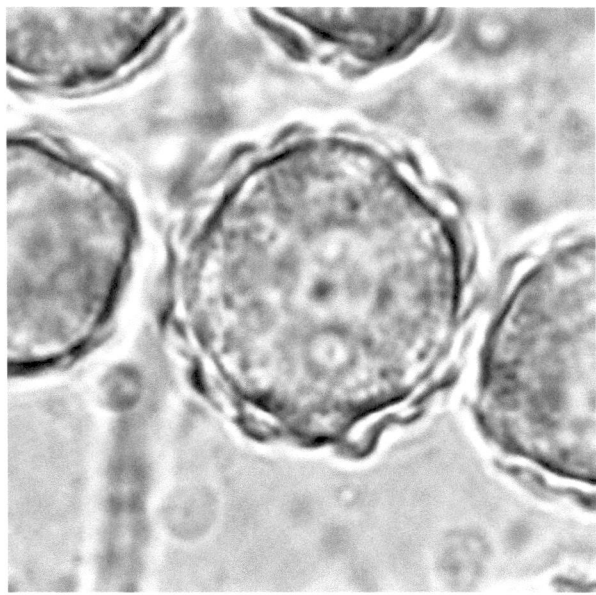

Fig. 2.14 Group II: the
average diameter of cysts
in this group is less than
18 μm (×1000)

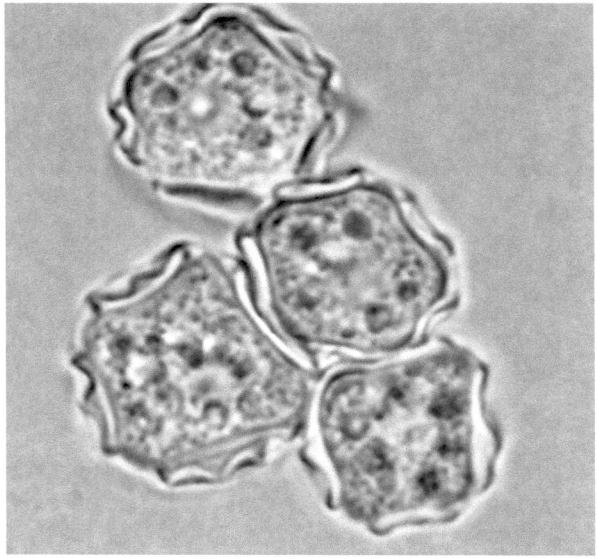

Group III: The average diameter of cysts is also less than 18 μm. The outer wall
is thin with or without wrinkles, and the inner wall is smooth with three to five
angles (Fig. 2.15). There are five species in group III, including *A. palestinen-
sis, A. culbertsoni, A. lenticulata, A. pustulosa, and A. royreba*.

Fig. 2.15 Group III: the outer wall of cyst is thin, and the inner wall of cyst is smooth (×1000)

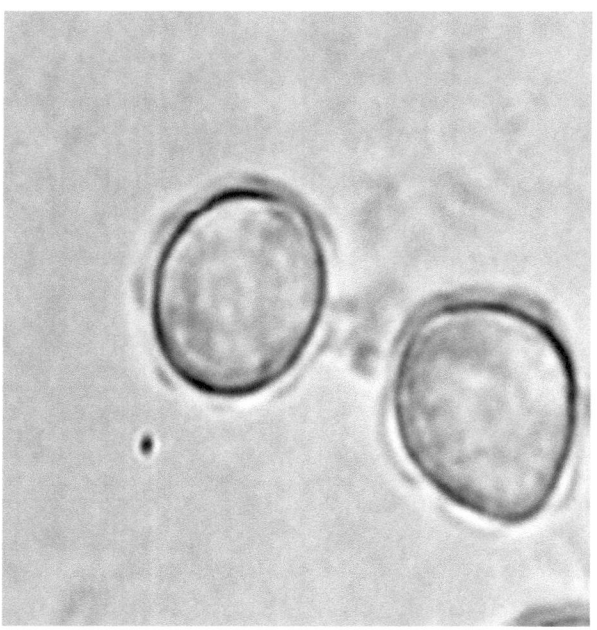

In 1991, *Visvesvara G.S.* added *A. tubiashi* in group I and *A. hatchetti* in group II into the classification of morphology [9]. The pathogenic *Acanthamoeba* mainly belongs to group II. Besides, *A. culbertsoni* of group III is also pathogenic [10].

- *Classification of Genotype*: Currently the most conventional classification scheme under the level of genus is based on the genotypes of *Acanthamoeba*. In other words, *Acanthamoeba* is categorized by the differences of DNA sequences among various strains belonging to the same genus. According to the most commonly used 18S rDNA genotyping, *Acanthamoeba* is subdivided into 19 genotypes, i.e., T_1–T_{19}.
- Among confirmed genotypes of *Acanthamoeba*, at least ten genotypes (including T_2, T_3, T_4, T_5, T_6, T_{10}, T_{11}, T_{13}, T_{15}, and T_{16}) were found to cause corneal infections in humans. Especially, genotype 4 (T_4) is the most frequently detected genotype that causes *Acanthamoeba* keratitis [11–13].

Yan Zhang et al. isolated *Acanthamoeba* strains from Chinese patients suffering from the keratitis and analyzed these strains with *18S rDNA* genotyping. They found that most of the pathogenic strains inducing the keratitis in China belonged to T_4 genotype, and occasionally T_3 genotype was isolated from very few cases [14]. In 2010, Lixin Xie et al. investigated the genotypes in 14 *Acanthamoeba* strains responsible for keratitis, and they found that all of isolated strains were T_4 genotype [15]. Table 2.2 reports the relationship between 18S rDNA sequence-based genotypes and groups categorized by morphology.

Table 2.2 Genotypes based on 18S rDNA sequence vs. morphology groups

Morphology groups	Genotypes
Group I	T7, T8, T9, T17
Group II, III	T1–T6, T10–T16

In 2014, Chao Jiang et al. in Beijing Institute of Ophthalmology identified genotypes of 100 *Acanthamoeba* strains that caused *Acanthamoeba* keratitis clinically. Out of 100 *Acanthamoeba* strains, 99 strains belonged to T_4 genotype (99%) and 1 strain to T_{11} (1%). Furthermore, a total of 27 subtypes were identified among the strains belonging to T_4 genotype, in which *subtypes* of $T_4/41$ and $T_4/31$ were most frequently detected. In addition, four novel T_4 subtypes that have not yet been reported in gene pool were detected and named as $T_4/42$, $T_4/43$, $T_4/44$, and $T_4/45$, respectively (in press).

Up to now, three genotypes of *Acanthamoeba*, i.e., T_4, T_{11}, and T_3, which caused keratitis, were reported in the Chinese mainland, and among these three genotypes, T_4 is the most common pathogenic genotype, and $T_4/41$ and $T_4/31$ are the most frequently identified subtypes.

- *Genotyping Methods*: The genotyping methods for *Acanthamoeba* that are currently applied are mainly as follows:
  1. *18S rDNA sequence typing*
  2. 2. *mtDNA*-restriction fragment length polymorphism (mtDNA-RFLP) typing

Because the method of whole rRNA 18S gene sequence typing is sophisticated and time-consuming, 18S rDNA sequence typing is applied more widely.

Booton et al. optimized the sequencing position of the JDP1-JDP2 PCR products to obtain a reliable and simplified genotyping method [16]. Loci 29 and 29-1 were detected in the sequence of PCR products through the amplification of *Acanthamoeba* 18S DNA (18S ribosomal RNA gene, *Rns*) by PCR primer JDP1-JDP2. Locus 29 is a highly conserved sequence, whereas locus 29-1 is frequently mutated. Currently, locus 29-1 is named as DF3 (Diagnosis Fragment 3) that provides information for genotype identification of *Acanthamoeba*.

Thus, the application of PCR amplification sequencing on the partial sequence of *Acanthamoeba* 18S rRNA that contains DF3 through specific primer JDP1-JDP2 is the most frequently used *Acanthamoeba* genotyping method [11].

2.2.4 Genotyping Identification of *Acanthamoeba* Strains in the Natural Environment

Acanthamoeba is widespread in the natural environment. The identification of *Acanthamoeba* genotypes enables us to trace the source of infectious pathogens and determine the risk factors of *Acanthamoeba* keratitis. The studies have reported that *Acanthamoeba* can be isolated from tap water, rivers, hot springs, soil, dust, air, and healthy and dead animals and frequently isolated strains of *Acanthamoeba* belonged to T_4 genotype [17–26].

In 2014, 42 samples from *tap water* and 30 samples from the *lake water* in Beijing districts were collected for the isolation of amoeba in Beijing Institute of Ophthalmology. After culture of amoeba for 14 days, the growth of amoeba was observed in 14 samples (33.3%) among the 42 tap water samples, and growth of amoeba was also detected in 14 samples (46.7%) among the 30 lake water samples.

PCR amplification sequencing was applied to amoeba strains by using universal amoeba primers, *Hartmannellidae-*, *Naegleria-*, and *Acanthamoeba*-specific primers, respectively. The results of sequencing showed that from tap water samples, eight strains belong to *Hartmannellidae*, and two strains belonged to *Naegleria* and *Acanthamoeba* (T_4 genotype), respectively. From lake water samples, 1 *Vahlkampfia* strain, 2 *Acanthamoeba* strains (T_4 genotype), and 11 *Hartmannellidae* strains were found. The results in this study indicated that amoeba existed in both tap water and lake water in Beijing districts. The most common isolated strains belonged to *Hartmannellidae*, followed by *Acanthamoeba*. Moreover, the positive isolated rate of amoeba from lake water samples was higher than that from tap water samples. Because tap water might be used abnormally for rinsing corneal contact lenses in some of the cases, it is considered as one of the risk factors which were related to *Acanthamoeba* keratitis in China.

In addition to morphological and genetic classification schemes, alternative methods such as the application of *isozymogram* or *monoclonal antibody* were also utilized to categorize *Acanthamoeba*. The analysis of these classifications provided the molecular biological basis for exploring the relationship between *Acanthamoeba* genotypes and pathogenicity as well as anti-amoeba drug sensitivity.

2.3   *Naegleria* spp.

Among *Naegleria* spp. that cause human diseases, *Naegleria fowleri* protozoa were extensively studied, which mainly infect the human central nervous system and subsequently cause fatal meningoencephalitis. However, a few cases of human corneal infections caused by *Naegleria fowleri* have been reported [4].

Naegleria fowleri is usually isolated from freshwater and exists in two forms, i.e., trophozoite and cyst in natural conditions. Different from *Acanthamoeba* spp., trophozoite of *Naegleria* spp. can transform into a third form (called as *flagellum*) in distilled water, which is an important biological characteristic structure in *differential diagnosis* for *etiology*.

2.3.1   Trophozoite

The size of *trophozoite of Naegleria fowleri* amoeba is relatively small with a diameter of 8–30 μm, and the trophozoite usually is round or oblong in shape. Its movement is active, but no spinous process is formed on the surface of the trophozoite. The characteristic morphological structure is the blunt round pseudopodium (also called as lobopodium).

Under light microscope, the cytoplasm of *Naegleria fowleri* trophozoite is granular and contains plenty of liquid vacuoles, contractile vacuoles, and food vacuoles.

A distinctive transparent nucleus can be observed in the cytoplasm, and a round dense porphyritic nucleolus is located in the center of the nucleus.

When the trophozoite is put into the distilled water for 2-h cultivation at a temperature of 37 °C, it can transform into a *piriform* flagellum. There are two or more (up to nine) *flagella* on one end of the cell. Flagellum can immigrate in the water. However, it neither regenerates itself by binary fission nor becomes cyst form. After around 24 h later, flagellum *transforms* back to trophozoite form again. Such temporary presence of flagellum can be regarded as an important biological feature that distinguishes *Naegleria* spp. from *Acanthamoeba* spp.

Under the *transmission electron microscope*, the cell membrane of *Naegleria fowleri* trophozoite is composed of two layers with high electron density materials and separated by a transparent area. The organelles in the cytoplasm arrange irregularly, and rough endoplasmic reticulum is in the shape of *long tubular vesicles* with ribosome attached to the surface. In addition, a large number of dumbbell-like mitochondria are observed in the cytoplasm. But typical Golgi apparatus can hardly be found. Liquid vacuoles, lysosomes, and food vacuoles containing *phagocytosis* and *cellular debris* can be observed in the cytoplasm. In lobopodium of trophozoite, there are no vesicles and glycogen and phospholipid particles. Two high electron density layers of nuclear membranes can be clearly detected around the nucleus with a dense *endosome* located at the center. In some strains of *Naegleria fowleri*, which are isolated from the lesion tissues of the patients, *red blood cells*, *white blood cells*, as well as some *virus-like particles* have been also found. Under scanning electron microscope, the surface of the cell membrane of trophozoite is irregular and consists of sucker-like structure (called as amebastome) that is related to the virulence, invasiveness, and phagocytic potency of *Naegleria* amoeba [3].

Trophozoite of *Naegleria fowleri* reproduces by binary fission that is characterized by typical mitosis. During prophase, the nucleus swells, and then the nucleolus is elongated till it is divided into two equivalent parts (known as polarization). At metaphase, the spindle is formed between the two polarized cytoplasms. Subsequently, during anaphase, chromatin is separated into two parts that further move to two polar regions, and polar caps disappear, but the nuclear membrane remains intact. During telophase, two *daughter nuclei* and then two daughter cells are formed.

Trophozoites of *Naegleria fowleri* are *heat-resistant* protozoa that can survive at a high temperature of up to 45 °C. Especially, they grow and reproduce with the highest speed rate at the temperature of 35 °C. Normally, the solution containing 10 ppm chlorine cannot kill *Naegleria fowleri* protozoa.

2.3.2 Cyst

Mature *cysts of Naegleria* spp. are relatively small in size and round in shape with a diameter of approximately 9 μm. Cysts consist of monolayer capsule wall that is usually smooth. On the surface of the cyst, there are one or two minute pore-like craters of volcanoes. The *pores* of *Naegleria fowleri* are flat. The cytoplasm of the cyst is finely granular with the nucleus located in the central area of the cyst. *Naegleria* cysts are also highly resistant to temperature and dryness like *Acanthamoeba* cysts. Cysts can transform into trophozoites through excysting from the pores of the wall under favorable conditions.

References

1. Zhang Y. Research advances in genotype and identification of *Acanthamoeba*. Section Ophthalmol Foreign Med Sci. 2002;26(4):214–7.
2. Marciano-Cabral F, Cabral G. *Acanthamoeba* spp. as agents of disease in humans. Clin Microbiol Rev. 2003;16(2):273–307.
3. Julio Martinez A. Free-living amebas: natural history, prevention, diagnosis, pathology, and treatment of disease. Boca Raton: CRC Press; 1985. p. 145–50.
4. Sun X, Jin X. *Acanthamoeba* keratitis. Ophthalmol CHN. 2002;11(1):4–6.
5. Auran JD, Starr MB, Jakobiec FA. *Acanthamoeba* keratitis. A review of the literature. Cornea. 1987;6(1):2–26.
6. Luo SY, Jin XY, Wang ZG, et al. Ultrastructure study of pathogen of *Acanthamoeba* keratitis. [Article in Chinese]. Zhonghua Yan Ke Za Zhi. 2008;44(11):1020–4.
7. Gao M, Zhang C, Yang X, et al. Influence of temperatures and pH value on biological activity of *Acanthamoeba* isolated from keratitis. Chin Ophthalmol Res. 2009;27(8):685–7.
8. Chen W, Sun X. Research advances in pathogenesis and immunological reactions for *Acanthamoeba* keratitis. Section Ophthalmol Foreign Med Sci. 2004;28(3):175–8.
9. Visvesvara GS. Classification of *Acanthamoeba*. Rev Infect Dis. 1991;13(Suppl 5):369–72.
10. Illingworth CD, Cook SD. *Acanthamoeba* keratitis. Surv Ophthalmol. 1998;42(6):493–508.
11. Magnet A, Henriques-Gil N, Galván-Diaz AL, et al. Novel *Acanthamoeba* 18S rRNA gene sequence type from an environmental isolate. Parasitol Res. 2014;113(8):2845–50.
12. Jiang C, Liang Q, Sun X. Genotyping of *Acanthamoeba* isolated from keratitis and clinical signification. Int Rev Ophthalmol. 2011;35(4):232–6.
13. Grun AL, Stemplewitz B, Scheid P. First report of an *Acanthamoeba* genotype T13 isolate as etiological agent of a keratitis in humans. Parasitol Res. 2014;113(6):2395–400.
14. Zhang Y, Sun X, Wang Z, et al. Identification of 18S ribosomal DNA genotype of *Acanthamoeba* from patients with keratitis in North China. Invest Ophthalmol Vis Sci. 2004;45(6):1904–7.
15. Zhao G, Sun S, Zhao J, et al. Genotyping of *Acanthamoeba* isolates and clinical characteristics of patients with *Acanthamoeba* keratitis in China. J Med Microbiol. 2010;59(Pt 4):462–6.
16. Booton GC, Kelly DJ, Chu YW, et al. 18S ribosomal DNA typing and tracking of *Acanthamoeba* species isolates from corneal scrape specimens, contact lenses, lens cases, and home water supplies of *Acanthamoeba* keratitis patients in Hong Kong. J Clin Microbiol. 2002;40(5):1621–5.
17. Abe N, Kimata I. Genotype of *Acanthamoeba* isolates from corneal scrapings and contact lens cases of *Acanthamoeba* keratitis patients in Osaka, Japan. Jpn J Infect Dis. 2010;63(4):299–301.
18. Nuprasert W, Putaporntip C, Pariyakanok L, et al. Identification of a novel t17 genotype of *Acanthamoeba* from environmental isolates and t10 genotype causing keratitis in Thailand. J Clin Microbiol. 2010;48(12):4636–40.
19. Huang SW, Hsu BM. Isolation and identification of *Acanthamoeba* from Taiwan spring recreation areas using culture enrichment combined with PCR. Acta Trop. 2010;115(3):282–7.
20. Niyyati M, Lorenzo-Morales J, Rahimi F, et al. Isolation and genotyping of potentially pathogenic *Acanthamoeba* strains from dust sources in Iran. Trans R Soc Trop Med Hyg. 2009;103(4):425–7.
21. Lorenzo-Morales J, Ortega-Rivas A, Martínez E, et al. *Acanthamoeba* isolates belonging to T1, T2, T3, T4 and T7 genotypes from environmental freshwater samples in the Nile Delta region, Egypt. Acta Trop. 2006;100(1-2):63–9.

22. De Jonckheere JF. Molecular identification of free-living amoebae of the Vahlkampfiidae and Acanthamoebidae isolated in Arizona (USA). Eur J Protistol. 2007;43(1):9–15.
23. Hsu B-M, Ma P-H, Liou T-S, et al. Identification of 18S ribosomal DNA genotype of *Acanthamoeba* from hot spring recreation areas in the central range, Taiwan. J Hydrol. 2009;367(3-4):249–54.
24. Niyyati M, Lorenzo-Morales J, Rezaie S, et al. Genotyping of *Acanthamoeba* isolates from clinical and environmental specimens in Iran. Exp Parasitol. 2009;121(3):242–5.
25. Lorenzo-Morales J, López-Darias M, Martínez-Carretero E, et al. Isolation of potentially pathogenic strains of *Acanthamoeba* in wild squirrels from the Canary Islands and Morocco. Exp Parasitol. 2007;117(1):74–9.
26. Rodriguez-Zaragoza S, Magana-Becerra A. Prevalence of pathogenic *Acanthamoeba* (Protozoa: Amoebidae) in the atmosphere of the city of San Luis Potosi, Mexico. Toxicol Ind Health. 1997;13(4):519–26.

Pathological Mechanisms and Immunological Reactions

3

3.1 Pathological Mechanisms

Acanthamoeba is a free-living amoeba whose natural host is not necessarily humans and is able to survive in the natural environment by feeding on bacteria, fungi, *algae*, and other protozoa. Therefore, about 25% of the trophozoites carry bacteria or other microbes. *Acanthamoeba* could also be isolated from the *throats* and *intestines* of *healthy people*. Human infections caused by pathogenic free-living amoeba such as *Acanthamoeba* keratitis usually result from an accidental contact or *opportunistic infections* [1].

As for corneal infection, *Acanthamoeba* protozoa first *adhere* to *lipopolysaccharide* or *mannosylated glycoproteins* on the corneal epithelial cell membranes followed by *phagocytosis* and *toxin* production. Subsequently, activated enzymes, such as neuraminidase, are released, leading to the thinning or death of the corneal epithelium cells and breach of the Bowman's membrane. Furthermore, the epithelial barrier function is destroyed so that *Acanthamoeba* protozoa can invade deep into the corneal stroma. *Acanthamoeba proteases* can destroy the collagens of the corneal *stroma*, and trophozoites can induce *radial keratoneuritis*.

Acanthamoeba protozoa damage the *barrier function* of the corneal epithelial layers through three ways: (a) in *endocytosis*, similar to the function of phagocytes, *Acanthamoeba* protozoa directly devour a part of the corneal cell membrane; (b) in *spontaneous exocytosis*, without the activation process, *Acanthamoeba* protozoa can release lysine spontaneously, which further damage the epithelial cell membrane; and (c) in *membrane-related activation* of exocytosis, when *Acanthamoeba* protozoa contact the surface of the corneal epithelium cells, the coalition on the membrane of the trophozoite can combine with the *receptor* or *ligand* on the surface of the *epithelial cell* membrane and further activates proteases, the release of which can result in the injury of the epithelial cells.

© Springer Nature Singapore Pte Ltd.
& People's Medical Publishing House, PR of China 2018
X. Sun, *Acanthamoeba Keratitis*, https://doi.org/10.1007/978-981-10-5212-5_3

3.1.1 Adhesive Attraction to the Corneal Epithelium

Acanthamoeba pathogenicity can be divided into two stages. At the first stage, trophozoites adhere to the corneal epithelium layer and cause the epithelial cell injury. Then the corneal lesions are mainly limited in the epithelial layer of the cornea. If adequate diagnosis and treatment is made at this stage, prognosis of the patients is often satisfactory clinically. At the second stage, trophozoites invade deep into the corneal stroma and reproduce themselves which can induce severe inflammation and damage to the corneal tissue.

The adhesive attraction of *Acanthamoeba* to the surface of the corneal epithelium is considered as the *initial stage* of the infection. Some studies reported that the adhesive attraction of *Acanthamoeba* to the cornea showed apparent *host specificity* [1, 2]. Panjwani et al. found that the adhesion potency of *Acanthamoeba* to human corneal epithelium is only 1.4 times stronger than that to rabbit corneal epithelium. It is experimentally proved that the adhesion potency of trophozoites to the cornea of rabbits is temperature-dependent. Between 25 °C and 35 °C, the adhesive attraction of *Acanthamoeba* to the corneal epithelium is relatively active and gradually enhances along with the increasing of temperature. A plateau occurs when the temperature reaches 35 °C. By contrast, no adhesion is observed when the temperature is 4 °C [3].

Complex *polysaccharides* on the surface of the corneal epithelial cell membrane are considered to be the adhesion locus of *Acanthamoeba* at early stage. In particular, *glycoproteins* and *glycolipids* make it easy for *Acanthamoeba* trophozoites to adhere to the surface of the corneal epithelium. Yang et al. discovered a protein, i.e., *mannose-connexin* with 136 KD molecular weight, expresses on the surface of *Acanthamoeba* membrane which can enhance the adhesive ability of *Acanthamoeba* to the corneal epithelial cells [4].

3.1.2 Non-contact Cytolysis Induced by Protease

The invasion of trophozoites to the corneal stroma may be related to a variety of proteases, including proteases with plenty of *serine, metalloproteinases, cysteine proteases, elastases, collagenases,* and specific *prothrombin activator*. However, the exact mechanism of these enzymes in the pathogenesis of the corneal infection by *Acanthamoeba* is still not clear [5, 6].

In vitro experiments have shown that trophozoites may release one type of *serine protease* with molecular weight of 100 KD when they were exposed to mannose for more than 48 h. This protease could induce in vitro non-contact cytolysis of the corneal epithelium. The potency of the proteases in pathogenic and nonpathogenic *Acanthamoeba* is different, i.e., *A. castellanii* (pathogenic strain), which can secrete plasma *zymogen activator* with molecular weight of 45–50 KD that makes it easy for trophozoites to invade into the corneal epithelium and stroma, but this activity is not found in nonpathogenic *Acanthamoeba* strains [7, 8].

3.1.3 Contact-Dependent Cytolysis

In addition to invading the corneal tissues through the action of proteases, *Acanthamoeba* can also damage the corneal epithelial cells by contact-dependent cytolysis. Although the mechanism of contact cytolysis still remains unclear, some of the studies have observed that the contact-dependent cytolysis was significantly enhanced if *dexamethasone* is added to the culture medium of the trophozoites and cysts of *Acanthamoeba*, and meantime trophozoites can also directly devour the corneal cells in the corneal stroma [9–12].

3.1.4 Apoptosis Mediated by *Acanthamoeba*

Experiments were conducted with cultured *monolayer fusion* of the human or rabbit corneal cells. The cysts of *Acanthamoeba* are able to transform into active trophozoites through excystation when the monolayer cells exist, which can further induce complete destruction of monolayer cells. It is suggested that such destructive effect is incubation time-dependent and related to the amount of *Acanthamoeba* pathogens. The trophozoites can induce the apoptosis of the corneal cells when pathogens invade into the corneal tissues. Accordingly, the apoptosis of the cells presents the *vacuoles* on the cell membrane, the increase of the *ratio of nucleus versus cytoplasm*, and *nucleosomes* forming. Additionally, DNA fragments with 180–200 bp are found.

With MTT method, the *cytotoxicity* induced by the trophozoites was observed when *Acanthamoeba* trophozoite was co-cultured with Hela cells. Hela cells showed typical apoptosis which was time-dependent. When B16 melanoma cells were used as target cells to study the cytotoxicity of *Acanthamoeba* trophozoites, it was shown that *B16 melanoma cells* displayed abnormal cellular adhesion to the culture dish and became round in shape after contacting with trophozoites. In addition, *vesicular protuberances* were generally found on the cell membranes along with the *pyknosis* of cell *nucleoplasm* that showed clustered distribution, which further led to apoptosis [13–16].

3.1.5 Cytokines

The corneal pathological research of *Acanthamoeba* keratitis demonstrated that in the first month of the corneal infection, the pathological changes of the corneal tissues were mainly necrosis and inflammatory cell infiltration, as shown in Fig. 3.1. There were plenty of *Acanthamoeba* pathogens in the corneal stroma, including the trophozoites with active proliferation ability and cysts at the stagnation stage of proliferation.

The expression of *matrix metalloproteinase 13* (MMP13) in the corneal tissues was intensively increased (Fig. 3.2). By contrast, the expression of *fibroblast growth factor 2* (FGF2) which is the maker of the repairing of the tissue was weakly positive. With the progression of the disease, *Acanthamoeba* could still be detected in the corneal tissues with disease duration from more than 1 month to half a year. Moreover, inflammatory

Fig. 3.1 *Acanthamoeba* keratitis for 1 month. The necrosis and inflammatory cell infiltration with a lot of *Acanthamoeba* pathogens in the tissues (HE-stained ×400)

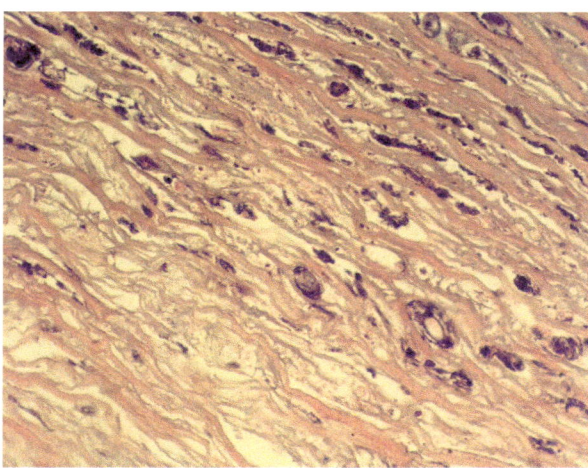

Fig. 3.2 *Acanthamoeba* keratitis for 1 month. The expression of MMP13 was strongly positive (×400)

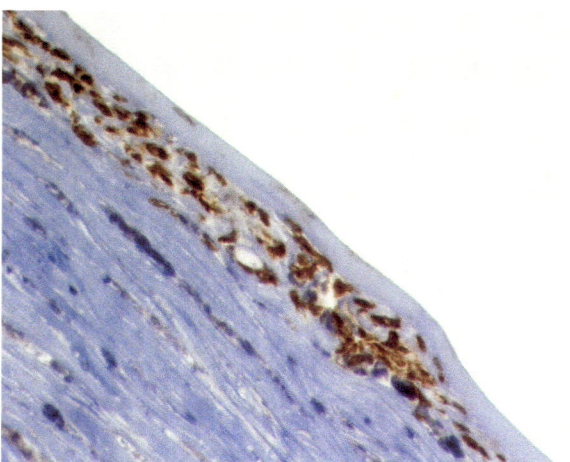

reactions within the corneal tissues also were obvious. The results of this study suggested that in clinical practice, the duration of anti-amoeba therapy generally might be required for more than half a year. Almost no inflammatory cell infiltration was observed in the corneal tissues with *anti-amoebic* treatment of more than 6 months, as shown in Fig. 3.3. The corneal stromal tissues began to repair. Neither cysts nor trophozoites were detected in the corneal stroma, and the expression of MMP13 in the corneal tissues was decreased, whereas the expression of FGF2 enhanced (Fig. 3.4). At same time, an abundance of *new vascular vessels* could be found in the corneal tissues [17].

Fig. 3.3 *Acanthamoeba* keratitis for 6 months. The corneal tissues began repair (HE-stained ×400)

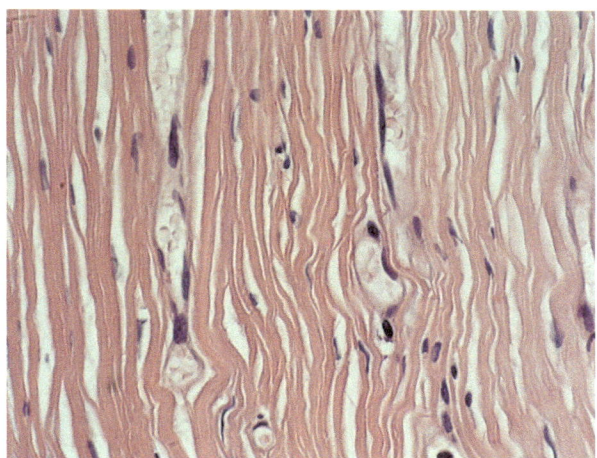

Fig. 3.4 *Acanthamoeba* keratitis for 6 months. The expression of FGF2 was positive (×400)

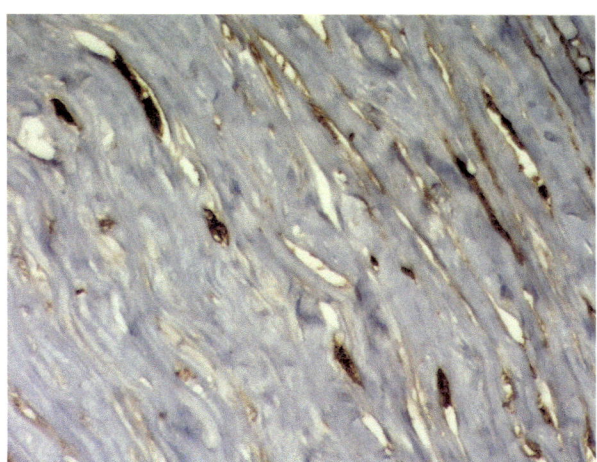

3.2   Immunological Reactions

Although the majority of healthy people have an encounter with *Acanthamoeba*, resulting in *humoral immune* responses in their body, and specific *anti-amoeba antibodies* can be found in the serum, only few people suffer from *Acanthamoeba* keratitis. The human body can have non-specific and specific immunoreactions to *Acanthamoeba* during infection.

3.2.1   Non-specific Immunoreaction

The normal cornea and conjunctiva have the protective *barrier function* to prevent the invasion of pathogenic microorganisms. Normal tears also contain a variety of *anti-pathogenic* microbial substances, such as *complement, immunoglobulin, bacteriolysin*, and *interferon* (IFN), which have the potency to dissolve and kill pathogenic microorganisms. Mononuclear phagocytes can directly devour pathogenic microorganisms in non-specific immune responses. Several in vitro experiments confirmed that *neutrophils* and *macrophages* could kill *Acanthamoeba* trophozoites with assistance of the specific antibodies. Furthermore, γ-IFN can enhance the phagocytosis of macrophages [18].

3.2.2   Specific Immunoreaction

The specific immunoreaction to *Acanthamoeba* mainly includes two types, i.e., humoral immunity and *cellular immunity*. Both of them also need the assistance of antigen-presenting cell.

3.2.2.1 Antigen-Presenting Cell

Langerhans cell (LC) is a type of antigen-presenting cell with high efficiency. The in vitro experiments found that the movement of Langerhans cells from the peripheral cornea toward the central area of the cornea can further accelerate specific delayed hypersensitivity and to some extent prevent the progression of *Acanthamoeba* keratitis. These effects might be related to the inhibition of the adhesion of the trophozoites to the corneal epithelial cells or the direct destruction of trophozoites by Langerhans cells [19, 20].

3.2.2.2 Humoral Immunity

Pathogenic free-living *Acanthamoeba* is widely distributed in nature. It has been shown that the positive rate of anti-amoeba antibody in the serum of healthy people is high. The antibodies are mainly *immunoglobulin G and M*, of which the titer ranges from 1:20 to 1:80. In addition, anti-*Acanthamoeba*-specific neutralizing agents are found in the serum. After the binding of specific antibodies to antigens on the surface of parasites, the complement system is activated in a classic pathway, leading to the dissolution of parasites. It was found in the in vitro experiments that *IgA* was produced after *Acanthamoeba* antigens were orally administered to Chinese hamsters. Although IgA did not influence the vitality of protozoa, it significantly inhibited the adhesion of protozoa to the corneal epithelial cell. The immunoreactivity of IgG and IgA in the serum of patients with *Acanthamoeba* keratitis was decreased significantly, and IgA in the serum lacks 29 KD and 47 KD bands, indicating that the humoral immune system of the patients had abnormal changes due to *Acanthamoeba* infection [21–23].

   Acanthamoeba can destroy the *immune effector* molecules in order to escape the immune responses of the host. Soluble metabolites and their complexes released by trophozoites can induce the changes in the morphology and function of human mononuclear cells. *Acanthamoeba* may induce apoptosis of host immune cells and stimulate the release of pro-inflammatory cytokines and proteinases which can further dissolve immunoglobulin. The release of protease *inhibitors* and other metabolites from *Acanthamoeba* can lead to the death of human *monocytes*, and the release of enzymes from *Acanthamoeba* can dissolve secreted immunoglobulin A (sIgA), IgG, and IgM. Moreover, the activity of these enzymes could not be inhibited by endogenous protease inhibitors from the host, and this enzyme even may be able to dissolve these *endogenous inhibitors*.

3.2.2.3 Cellular Immunity

Ring infiltration (RI) of the cornea is the most characteristic clinical sign during the course of *Acanthamoeba* keratitis and is a type of cellular immunoreaction associated with the invasion of *Acanthamoeba* in the *subepithelium* or the stroma. It was confirmed that the antigens of *Acanthamoeba* could dramatically enhance the proliferation for human peripheral blood T lymphocytes. *Acanthamoeba* cysts exhibit *antigenicity* and immunogenicity simultaneously and can induce cellular immune responses of the host. It was reported that T lymphocytes within the spleen tissues showed proliferative reaction after mice were immunized by the antigens of cysts. However, such reaction was not observed if mice were immunized by the antigens of trophozoites. It implied that the antigens of trophozoites might be able to inhibit the cell-mediated immune responses, which could also reflect the clinical pathological finding that *lymphocyte* infiltrations in the corneal tissues were rather limited when trophozoites were mainly found in the corneal stroma at the early stage of disease [24, 25].

Since *Acanthamoeba* is able to escape from the killing of immune system of the host, they may stay in infected tissues for a long time (from several months to several years). A research reported that *Acanthamoeba* cysts could survive in the corneal tissues for up to 31 months, and its antigens remained even longer in the corneal tissues, which could induce protracted course of the keratitis and even the *scleral* inflammations. It was observed in some of the clinical cases of *Acanthamoeba* keratitis that the continuous inflammatory reactions at late stage might be related to the immunoreaction to parasite antigens [26].

3.2.3 Preventive Immunoreaction

Acanthamoeba keratitis may relapse during the treatment, indicating that patients have not set up the persistent *acquired immunity*. The oral application of *Acanthamoeba* antigens (mixed with cholera toxin) to immunize animals can significantly reduce the infection rate of *Acanthamoeba*. Specific anti-amoeba antibody IgA can be detected in the mucosa, feces, and tears of animals that were immunized by orally feeding *Acanthamoeba* antigens. Based on the results of the experiments in which pigs were immunized by oral *Acanthamoeba* antigens, although large amounts of Th1 cells and serum IgG antibodies were detected in the immunized animals, *Acanthamoeba* keratitis could not be entirely prevented. By contrast, through the subconjunctival injection of *Acanthamoeba* antigens with the same dosage by oral, effective immunity against *Acanthamoeba* keratitis was observed only in 50% of the immunized animals. It is suggested that the *conjunctiva-associated lymphoid tissue* (CALT) was activated in which an abundance of mucosal secreting IgA was produced through the classic pathway and the adhesion of *Acanthamoeba* to the corneal epithelial cells was inhibited. Accordingly, *Acanthamoeba* keratitis might be prevented [27–29].

References

1. Niederkorn JY, Alizadeh H, Leher H, et al. The pathogenesis of *Acanthamoeba* keratitis. Microbes Infect. 1999;1(6):437–43.
2. Niederkorn JY, Ubelaker JE, McCulley JP, et al. Susceptibility of corneas from various animal species to in vitro binding and invasion by *Acanthamoeba castellanii* [corrected]. Invest Ophthalmol Vis Sci. 1992;33(1):104–12.
3. Panjwani N, Zhao Z, Baum J, et al. *Acanthamoebae* bind to rabbit corneal epithelium in vitro. Invest Ophthalmol Vis Sci. 1997;38(9):1858–64.
4. Yang Z, Cao Z, Panjwani N. Pathogenesis of *Acanthamoeba* keratitis: carbohydrate-mediated host-parasite interactions. Infect Immun. 1997;65(2):439–45.
5. Kay EP, He YG. Post-transcriptional and transcriptional control of collagen gene expression in normal and modulated rabbit corneal endothelial cells. Invest Ophthalmol Vis Sci. 1991;32(6):1821–7.
6. Larkin DF, Easty DL. External eye flora as a nutrient source for *Acanthamoeba*. Graefes Arch Clin Exp Ophthalmol. 1990;228(5):458–60.
7. Mitra MM, Alizadeh H, Gerard RD, et al. Characterization of a plasminogen activator produced by *Acanthamoeba castellanii*. Mol Biochem Parasitol. 1995;73(1-2):157–64.
8. Khan NA, Jarroll EL, Panjwani N, et al. Proteases as markers for differentiation of pathogenic and nonpathogenic species of *Acanthamoeba*. J Clin Microbiol. 2000;38(8):2858–61.
9. McClellan K, Howard K, Niederkorn JY, et al. Effect of steroids on *Acanthamoeba* cysts and trophozoites. Invest Ophthalmol Vis Sci. 2001;42(12):2885–93.
10. Park DH, Palay DA, Daya SM, et al. The role of topical corticosteroids in the management of *Acanthamoeba* keratitis. Cornea. 1997;16(3):277–83.
11. John T, Lin J, Sahm D, et al. Effects of corticosteroids in experimental *Acanthamoeba* keratitis. Rev Infect Dis. 1991;13(Suppl 5):S440–2.
12. Pettit DA, Williamson J, Cabral GA, et al. In vitro destruction of nerve cell cultures by *Acanthamoeba* spp.:a transmission and scanning electron microscopy study. J Parasitol. 1996;82(5):769–77.
13. Larkin DF, Berry M, Easty DL. In vitro corneal pathogenicity of *Acanthamoeba*. Eye (Lond.). 1991;5(Pt 5):560–8.
14. Alizadeh H, Pidherney MS, McCulley JP, et al. Apoptosis as a mechanism of cytolysis of tumor cells by a pathogenic free-living amoeba. Infect Immun. 1994;62(4):1298–303.
15. An Q, Zhang X, Mei B, et al. Cytotoxic effect of *Acanthamoeba* trophozoite on hela cells. Chin J Parasitol Parasit Dis. 2001;19(1):37–40.
16. An Q, Zheng Y, Zhang P, et al. Cytotoxic effect of *Acanthamoeba* trophozoites on human melanoma cells. Acta Parasitol Med Entomol Sin. 2002;9(1):7–11.
17. Chen W, Sun X, Liang Q, et al. The clinical and histopathologic changes of experimental *Acanthamoeba* keratitis in rabbit. Chin Ophthalmic Res. 2009;27(1):27–31.

18. Stewart GL, Kim I, Shupe K, et al. Chemotactic response of macrophages to *Acanthamoeba castellanii* antigen and antibody-dependent macrophage-mediated killing of the parasite. J Parasitol. 1992;78(5):849–55.
19. van Klink F, Leher H, Jager MJ, et al. Systemic immune response to *Acanthamoeba* keratitis in the Chinese hamster. Ocul Immunol Inflamm. 1997;5(4):235–44.
20. van Klink F, Alizadeh H, He Y, et al. The role of contact lenses, trauma, and Langerhans cells in a Chinese hamster model of *Acanthamoeba* keratitis. Invest Ophthalmol Vis Sci. 1993;34(6):1937–44.
21. Cursons RT, Brown TJ, Keys EA, et al. Immunity to pathogenic free-living amoebae: role of humoral antibody. Infect Immun. 1980;29(2):401–7.
22. Walochnik J, Obwaller A, Haller-Schober EM, et al. Anti-*Acanthamoeba* IgG, IgM, and IgA immunoreactivities in correlation to strain pathogenicity. Parasitol Res. 2001;87(8):651–6.
23. Mattana A, Cappai V, Alberti L, et al. ADP and other metabolites released from *Acanthamoeba castellanii* lead to human monocytic cell death through apoptosis and stimulate the secretion of proinflammatory cytokines. Infect Immun. 2002;70(8):4424–32.
24. Bingji S, He X, Zhu L, et al. The clinical value of annular infiltration in the diagnosis and treatment of Acanthamoeba keratitis. American Medical Association. J Ophthalmol. 2000;12:40–2.
25. McClellan K, Howard K, Mayhew E, et al. Adaptive immune responses to *Acanthamoeba* cysts. Exp Eye Res. 2002;75(3):285–93.
26. Yang YF, Matheson M, Dart JK, et al. Persistence of *Acanthamoeba* antigen following *Acanthamoeba* keratitis. Br J Ophthalmol. 2001;85(3):277–80.
27. Leher HF, Alizadeh H, Taylor WM, et al. Role of mucosal IgA in the resistance to *Acanthamoeba* keratitis. Invest Ophthalmol Vis Sci. 1998;39(13):2666–73.
28. Alizadeh H, He Y, McCulley JP, et al. Successful immunization against *Acanthamoeba* keratitis in a pig model. Cornea. 1995;14(2):180–6.
29. Niederkorn JY. The role of the innate and adaptive immune responses in *Acanthamoeba* keratitis. Arch Immunol Ther Exp. 2002;50(1):53–9.

4.1   General Conditions

Patients with *Acanthamoeba* keratitis usually are healthy people. Any age may be affected. The population of male and female patients is almost equivalent. The majority of patients are infected unilaterally. Infection with *Acanthamoeba* in both eyes is not usually observed [1].

4.1.1   Distribution Characteristics of Ages

Between May 1991 and July 2014, a total of *267* cases were diagnosed as *Acanthamoeba* keratitis (with the corneal scrapping and/or cultivation of *Acanthamoeba* and/or corneal confocal microscopy) by the Department of Ocular Microbiology in *Beijing Institute of Ophthalmology (BIO)*. According to the statistical results on these data, the ages of patients ranged from 7 years to 82 years, with the average of 42 years and standard deviation of 14 years. The detailed distribution of patients over different age groups is reported in Table 4.1.

Table 4.1 Age distribution of 267 patients with *Acanthamoeba* keratitis

Age	No. of cases	Percentage (%)
–14	6	2.2
15–30	64	24.0
31–60	169	63.3
61–	28	10.5
Total	267	100.0

© Springer Nature Singapore Pte Ltd.
& People's Medical Publishing House, PR of China 2018
X. Sun, *Acanthamoeba Keratitis*, https://doi.org/10.1007/978-981-10-5212-5_4

Table 4.2 Gender distribution of 267 patients with *Acanthamoeba* keratitis

Gender	No. of cases	Percentage (%)
Male	151	56.6
Female	116	43.4
Total	267	100.0

4.1.2 Distribution Characteristics of Genders

No gender predilection has been noted. From the data of BIO, among 267 patients with *Acanthamoeba* keratitis, the ratio of male vs. female is 1.30:1. Hence, the proportion of male patients is slightly higher than female patients, as illustrated in Table 4.2.

4.1.3 Distribution Characteristics of Occupations

The distribution of occupations was analyzed for a series of 194 patients with *Acanthamoeba* keratitis in BIO. It has been shown that patients were mainly engaged in four kinds of occupations, i.e., approximately 50.0% of the patients were farm workers, 23.7% students, 10.3% office clerks, and 8.8% factory workers. It is noteworthy that there were four patients who were medical personnel, two of them were suspected to be infected during the clinical work in hospital [2, 3], as listed in Table 4.3.

4.1.4 Risk Factors

Acanthamoeba keratitis is generally associated with risk factors, such as contact lenses wear, trauma, etc. In *developed countries*, the primary risk factor was found to be contact lenses wear. In China, the most common risk factor is trauma, followed by corneal contact lenses wear. To characterize the distribution of risk factors in patients suffering from *Acanthamoeba* keratitis, BIO investigated the risk factors in a series of 182 patients in detail. Among the common risk factors, trauma was most frequently observed (accounting for 53.8%), followed by corneal contact lenses wear (29.1%), as reported in Table 4.4.

Analysis of the data in 182 cases of *Acanthamoeba* keratitis shows that in farm worker patients the major risk factor is trauma while that in student patients usually is contact lenses wear or orthokeratology (OK) lenses in China.

Most of the patients with *Acanthamoeba* keratitis associated with vegetal traumas are infected in accidental scratches on the cornea by leaves and stems (such as corn, wheat, rice and tree branches and leaves of fruits, etc.) during agricultural labor without appropriated eye protection, while other traumas which are related to *Acanthamoeba* keratitis mainly include sewage pollution, splash of winged insects, and wiping eyes with items that are contaminated with pathogen.

Table 4.3 Occupational distribution of 194 patients with *Acanthamoeba* keratitis

Occupation	No. of cases	Percentage (%)
Farm worker	97	50.0
Student	46	23.7
Office clerk	20	10.3
Factory worker	17	8.8
Medical personnel	4	2.1
Other	10	5.2
Total	194	100.0

Table 4.4 Distribution of risk factors in 182 Cases of *Acanthamoeba* keratitis

Risk factor	No. of cases	Percentage (%)
Trauma	98	53.8
Vegetal trauma	35	19.2
Non-vegetal other traumas	63	34.6
Corneal contact lenses wear	53	29.1
Medical history of keratitis	8	4.4
Other	23	12.6
Total	182	100.0

Contact lenses include soft corneal contact lenses, rigid gas permeable contact lenses, orthokeratology (OK) contact lenses, etc. Other traumas include foreign matters such as iron filings and coal cinders entering eyes and contaminated water, winged insects, or dust splashing into eyes

Table 4.5 Seasonal distribution of the morbidity among 267

Season	No. of cases	Percent (%)
Spring (March to June)	65	24.3
Summer (June to Sep.)	81	30.3
Autumn (Sep. to Dec.)	63	23.6
Winter (Dec. to March)	58	21.7
Total	267	100.0

Cases of *Acanthamoeba* keratitis in BIO

4.1.5 Seasonal Morbidity

The analysis on seasonal morbidity of 267 cases of *Acanthamoeba* keratitis showed that the seasonal characteristics of the morbidity of this disease are not obvious. Just in the summer, the number of patients infected is slightly higher than that in other three seasons, as reported in Table 4.5.

4.2 Clinical Symptoms

Compared with acute suppurative bacterial keratitis, the onset of *Acanthamoeba* keratitis is generally *chronic* and sometime *indolent*, which takes about 3–7 days after exposure to risk factors. Most of the patients are unilaterally infected. Out of

267 cases of *Acanthamoeba* keratitis investigated in BIO, 266 cases were induced by *infections unilaterally*, i.e., accounting for 99.6%, whereas only 1 patient (0.4%) suffered from infections in both eyes. Some of literatures reported that *Acanthamoeba* keratitis was *bilateral* in 10.8–11% of patients in the USA [4, 5]. This difference may be resulted from different primary risk factor, which is contact lens wear in the USA, correspondingly trauma being primary risk factor in China.

At the beginning of *onset of disease*, patients only present with mild, less characteristic symptoms, such as *eye discomfort*, mild *foreign body sensation*, moderate red eyes, etc. Meanwhile, the *vision acuity* is generally not significantly affected or just mild loss of vision acuity. Hence, most patients either would not go to see a doctor timely or are often misdiagnosed as viral keratitis, subsequently receiving viral keratitis treatment, some of cases also with the use of corticosteroids.

With the progression of the disease if misdiagnosis or delay diagnosis, severer symptoms may present intensively apparent, including *photophobia*, *lacrimation*, *ophthalmalgia*, and *blurred vision*. In addition, severe ophthalmalgia was observed in a number of patients, and the magnitude of such pain was not proportional to the degree of severity of corneal signs, which is also termed as "*the discrepancy* between symptoms and signs." Among 20 cases of *Acanthamoeba* keratitis analyzed in 1 study, 11 cases (i.e., 55%) displayed the symptom of severe ophthalmalgia [6]. During the treatment, some patients may have severe headache, orbital pain, nausea, and so on, which may be due to increased intraocular pressure, severe *limbitis* or *scleritis*, severe radial keratoneuritis, intensive anterior chamber inflammation, and toxicity of anti-*Acanthamoeba* eye drop.

4.3   Clinical Signs

Clinical signs of *Acanthamoeba* keratitis can be divided into three different phases according to the degree of infective severity: early stage, advanced stage, and later stage [7], and worthwhile notice that classification of clinical signs may not be consistent with the reported duration of disease.

4.3.1   Early Stage

At early stage, patients usually have the lesions located in corneal epithelium and shallow corneal stroma with the following manifestations: ocular *ciliary congestion*, *roughness* of corneal epithelium, corneal *epithelial punctate opacity*, subepithelial *infiltration*, or recurrent *epithelial erosion*. Occasionally, the infiltration may involve in the anterior third of the corneal stoma (as exemplified in Figs. 4.1, 4.2, 4.3, and 4.4).

A few of patients may have the presentations of the *pseudodendrites* of corneal epithelium or *disciform-like corneal edema*. The pseudodendrites of corneal epithelium is characterized by fine but few branches without swelling at the end of the branches. In addition, the branch edge region rarely yields dye penetration when *fluorescein staining*; see Figs. 4.5, 4.6, and 4.7.

Fig. 4.1 A female patient, 30 years old, SCL medical history, *Acanthamoeba* keratitis with corneal epithelium opacity

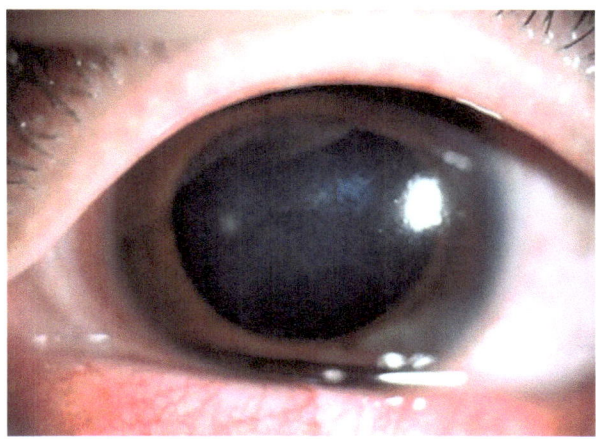

Fig. 4.2 A male patient, 37 years old, was hurt by maize leaf scratch for a half month, *Acanthamoeba* keratitis with corneal subepithelial infiltration

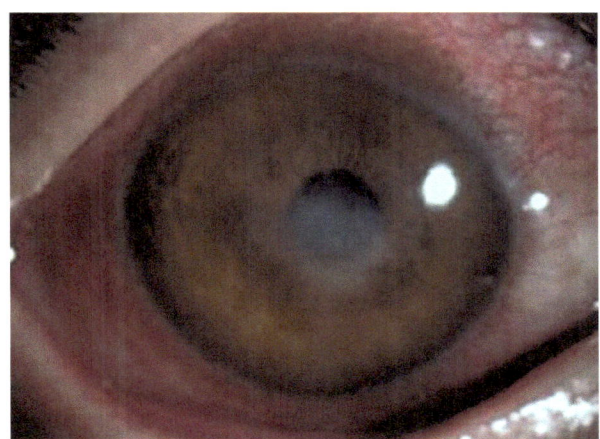

Fig. 4.3 A female patient, 17 years old, SCL history, *Acanthamoeba* keratitis with corneal epithelium edema and infiltration of shallow stroma

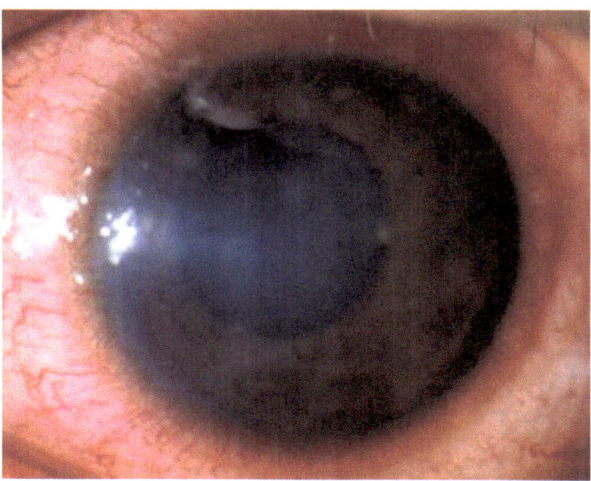

Fig. 4.4 A female patient, 20 years old, SCL, *Acanthamoeba* keratitis with corneal epithelium edema and maculosus infiltration of shallow stroma

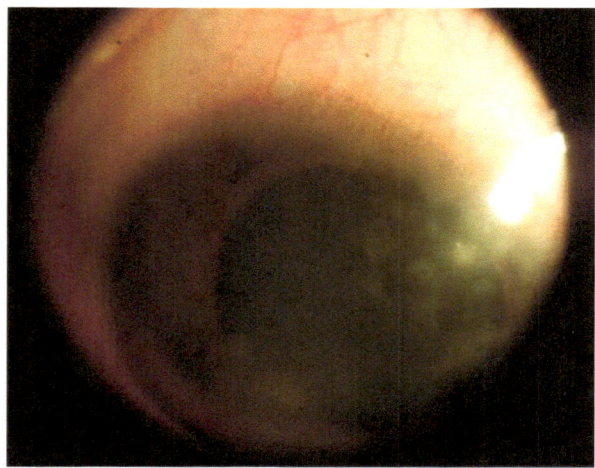

Fig. 4.5 A male patient, 20 years old, with history of OK contact lenses wear, bilateral *Acanthamoeba* keratitis for 15 days, with pseudodendrites on the corneal epithelium of (hollow arrow), accompanied by radial keratoneuritis (solid arrow)

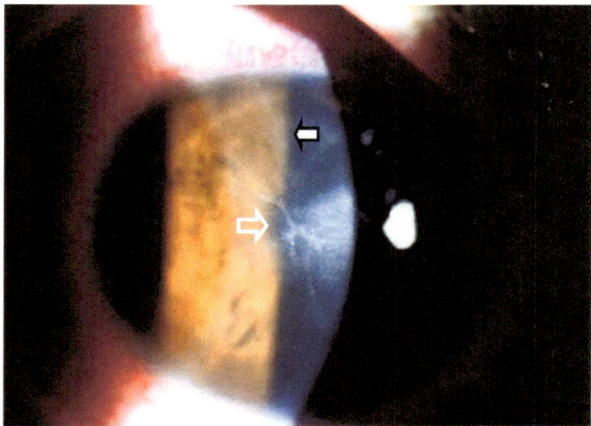

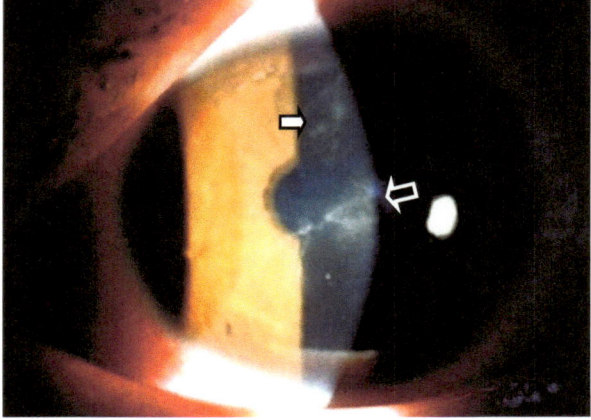

Fig. 4.6 A female patient,
13 years old, history of OK
contact lens wear,
Acanthamoeba keratitis
with disciform-like corneal
edema

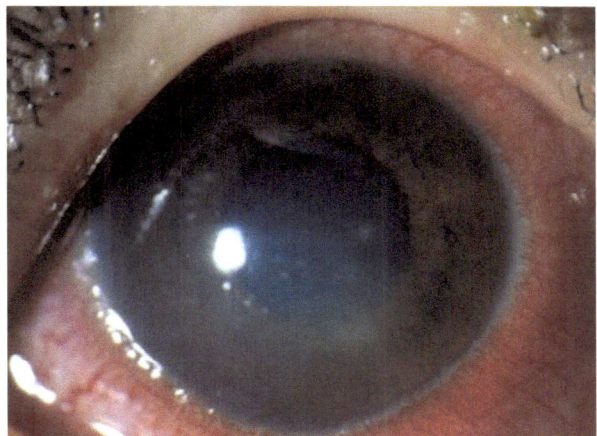

Fig. 4.7 A patient was
32 years old
Acanthamoeba keratitis
with disciform-like corneal
edema

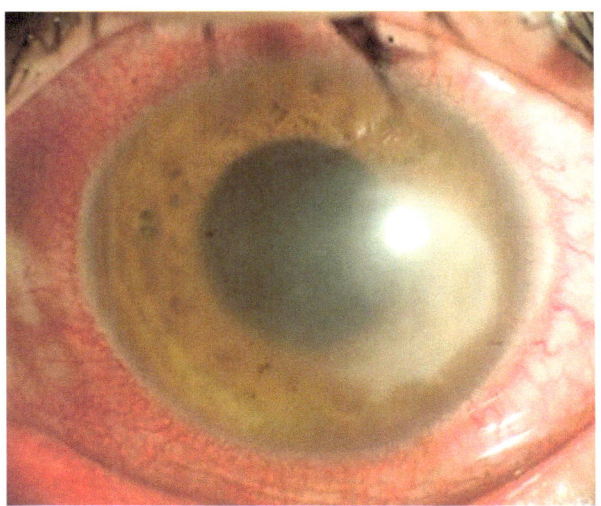

At early stage, some of patients may also have corneal *anterior stromal ulcer* usually with a diameter of less than 4 mm, shown in Figs. 4.8 and 4.9. Radial keratoneuritis is considered as the characteristic manifestation of early stage of the disease of *Acanthamoeba* keratitis (see Figs. 4.10 and 4.11). The data from a previous study by BIO showed that the incidence rate of *radial keratoneuritis* is only *10%* [8].

Acanthamoeba keratitis at early stage is usually misdiagnosed as herpes simplex virus infection [3]. For the majority of patients, corneal lesions may be transiently improved with the treatment of antivirus medicine and corticosteroids. However, after that, the corneal lesions of the patients may suffer a *relapse* soon with a repeated and aggravating tendency. With inappropriate treatments

Fig. 4.8 A female patient, 24 years old, the experience of OK contact lenses wear, *Acanthamoeba* keratitis with corneal superficial stromal ulcer

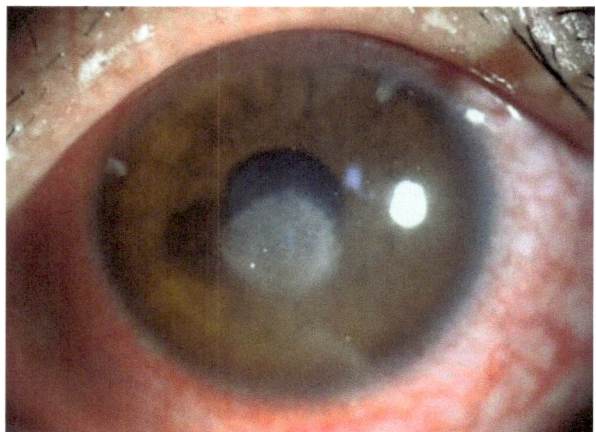

Fig. 4.9 A male patient, 43 years old, *Acanthamoeba* keratitis with corneal superficial stromal ulcer

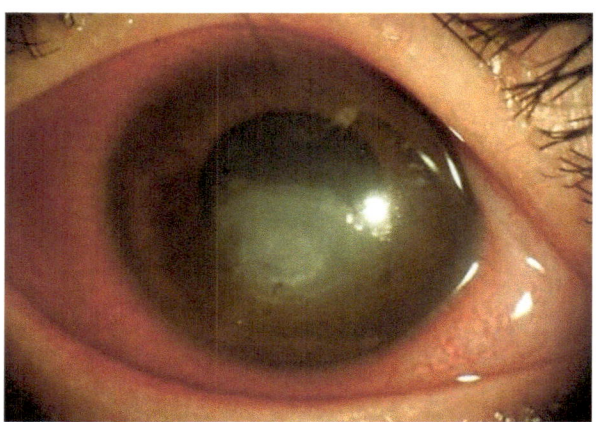

Fig. 4.10 A male patient, 16 years old, *Acanthamoeba* keratitis with corneal superficial stromal ulcer that was accompanied by radial keratoneuritis (shown by arrow)

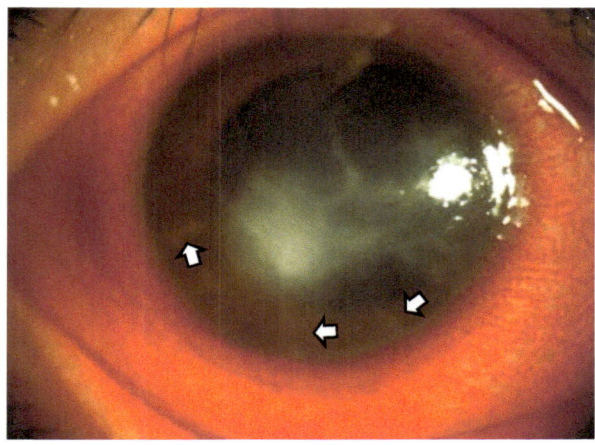

Fig. 4.11 A female
patient, 52 years old,
Acanthamoeba keratitis
corneal superficial stromal
ulcer that was
accompanied by radial
keratoneuritis (shown by
arrow)

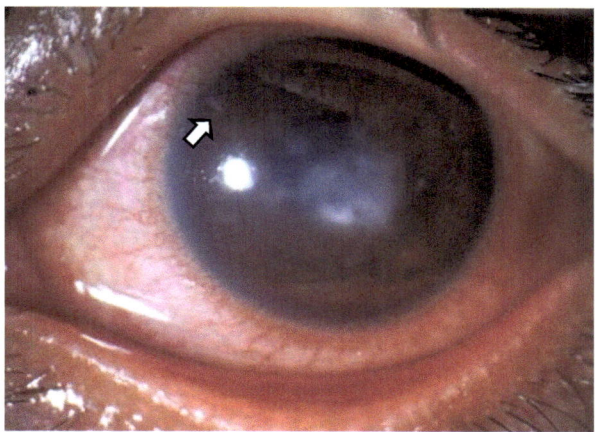

of corticosteroids eye drops or subconjunctival injection of corticosteroids for a
period of time, corneal infiltration or *ulceration* may aggravate abruptly, forming a large area of *deep stromal ulcer* with severe *hypopyon*, even *perforation* of
the cornea.

4.3.2 Advanced Stage

At this stage the lesion of the cornea may not restrict to the epithelium or shallow
corneal stroma. Most of patients have deep corneal *stromal ulcer* with a diameter
of generally larger than 5 mm at the central or eccentric corneal area. The ulceration of the cornea does not have a clear boundary and the surface of the ulcer has
hoary infiltration. In some of severe cases, even *necrotic tissues* and purulent
discharges on the surface of the corneal ulcer are observed. More compact infiltration is often observed in the *peripheral area* of the corneal ulcer than that of the
central area. Furthermore, on the edge of the ulcer, epithelial and subepithelial
compact infiltration that presents crude punctative and *salt-like* with slight protuberance can be observed. *Ditch-shaped melting* in the marginal zone of the corneal ulcer is a common corneal sign in severe cases. Four patients at advanced
stage with varying manifestations are presented in Figs. 4.12, 4.13, 4.14, and 4.15.

At advanced stage, the corneal ring infiltration was found in some of cases,
revealing an incidence rate of 28.6% [9], as exemplified in Figs. 4.16 and 4.17. In
ring infiltration area, the corneal epithelium could be complete or have epithelium
defect or stromal ulcer, as shown in Figs. 4.18 and 4.19.

The *ring corneal infiltration* may be of a complete or an *incomplete single ring*
(Fig. 4.20) but also be of *double concentric rings* (Fig. 4.21). A number of the patients
with the ring infiltration also have hypopyon, as reported in Figs. 4.22 and 4.23.

Fig. 4.12 *Acanthamoeba* keratitis at advanced stage, with the corneal stromal ulcer, more compact the infiltration in the peripheral area, ditch-shaped melting in peripheral the area of the corneal ulcer

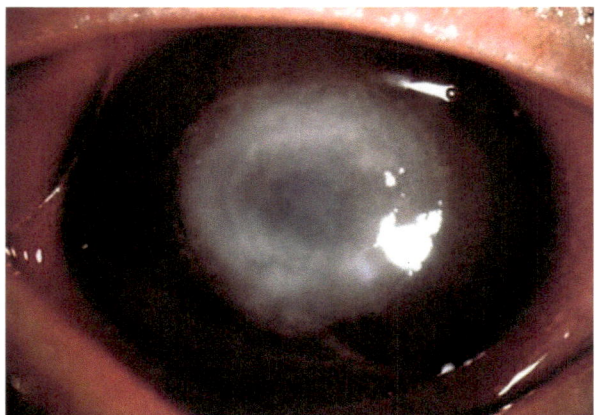

Fig. 4.13 *Acanthamoeba* keratitis at advanced stage, with the corneal stromal ulcer, and ditch-shaped melting in the peripheral area of the cornea

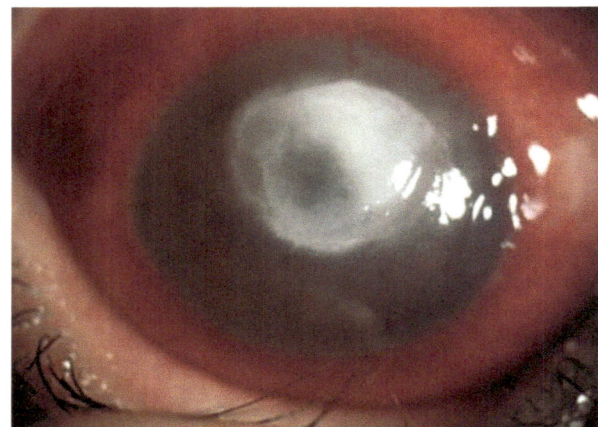

Fig. 4.14 *Acanthamoeba* keratitis at advanced stage, with subepithelial compact infiltrations in the peripheral area of ulcers, ditch-shaped melting in the peripheral area of the corneal ulcer (as shown by the arrow)

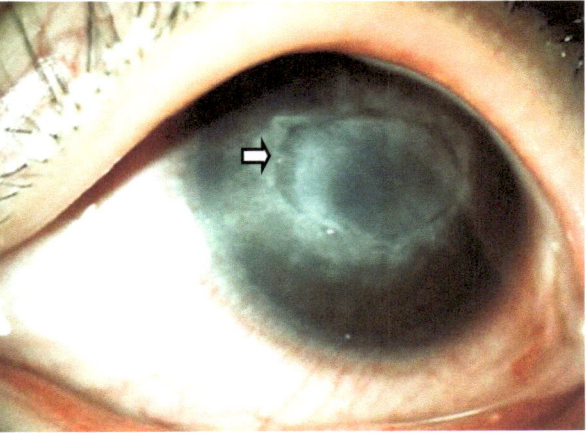

Fig. 4.15 *Acanthamoeba* keratitis at advanced stage, with subepithelial compact infiltrations in the peripheral area of ulcers. In addition, ditch-shaped melting is observed in the peripheral area of the corneal ulcer (as shown by the arrow)

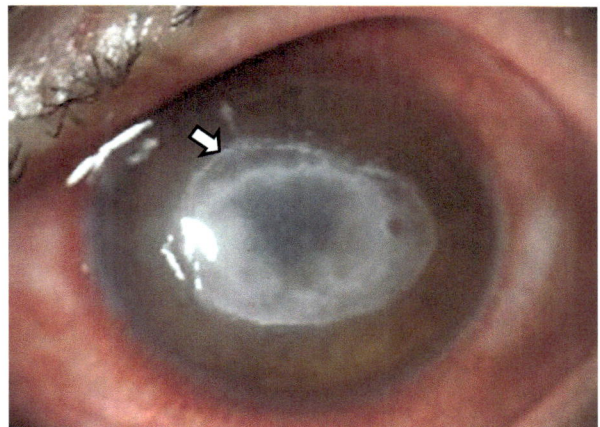

Fig. 4.16 *Acanthamoeba* keratitis at advanced stage, with moderate ring corneal infiltration and stroma edema without overlying epithelium defect

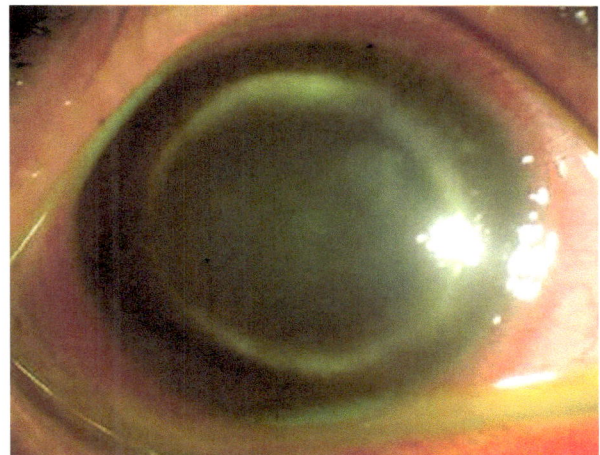

Fig. 4.17 *Acanthamoeba* keratitis at advanced stage, with severe ring corneal infiltration without overlying epithelium defect

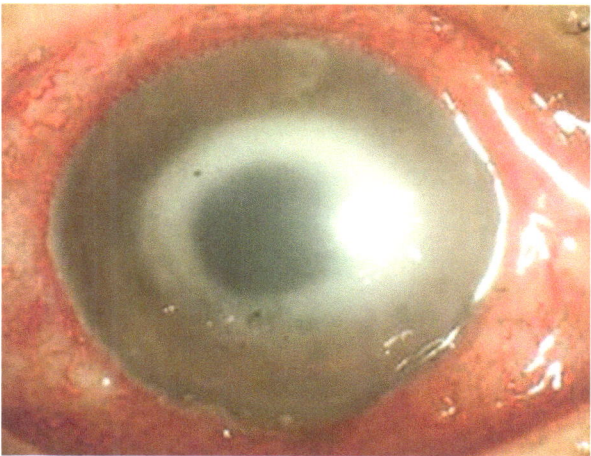

Fig. 4.18 *Acanthamoeba* keratitis at advanced stage, with ring corneal infiltration and moderate stroma edema with overlying epithelium defect

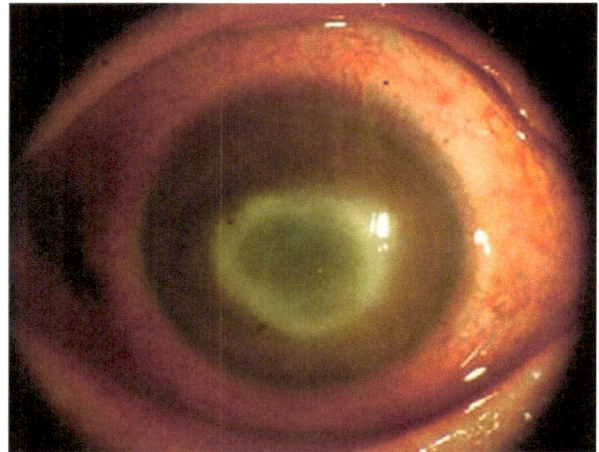

Fig. 4.19 *Acanthamoeba* keratitis at advanced stage, with ring corneal infiltration and moderate stroma edema with overlying epithelium and shallow stromal ulcer, positive fluorescein staining

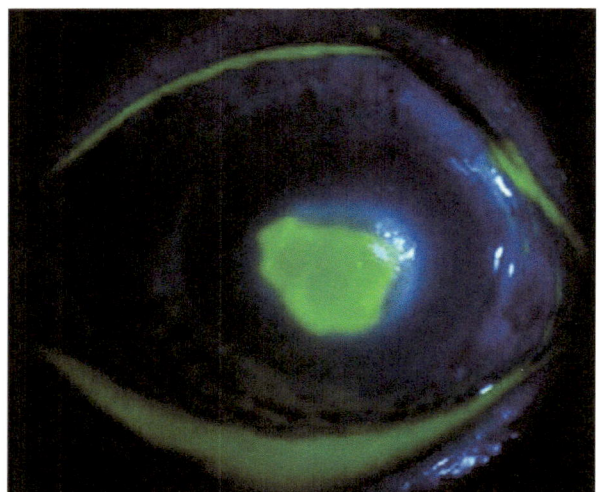

Fig. 4.20 *Acanthamoeba* keratitis at advanced stage, with incomplete ring corneal infiltration and moderate stroma edema with hypopyon

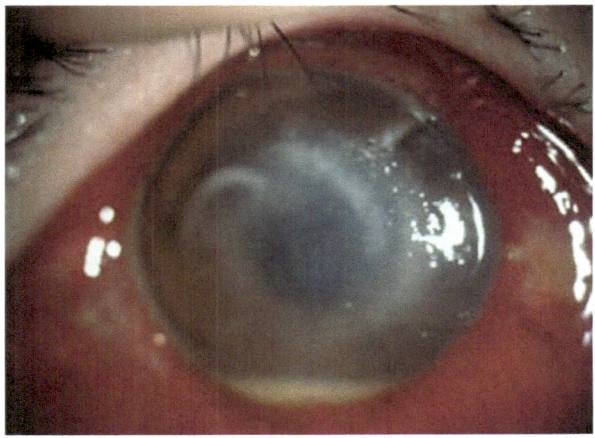

Fig. 4.21 *Acanthamoeba* keratitis at advanced stage, with double ring corneal infiltration and severe stroma edema

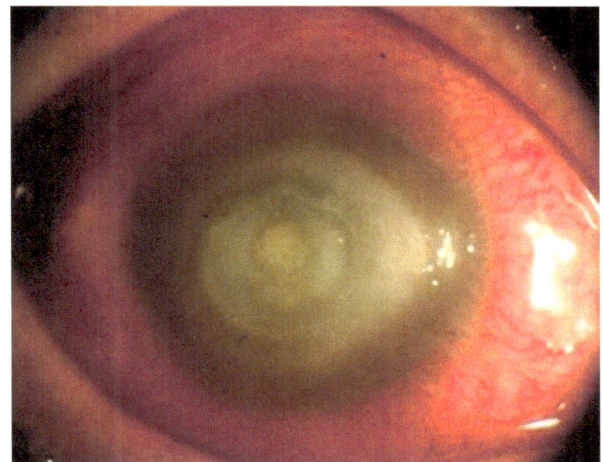

Fig. 4.22 *Acanthamoeba* keratitis at advanced stage, with stromal ulcer accompanied by hypopyon

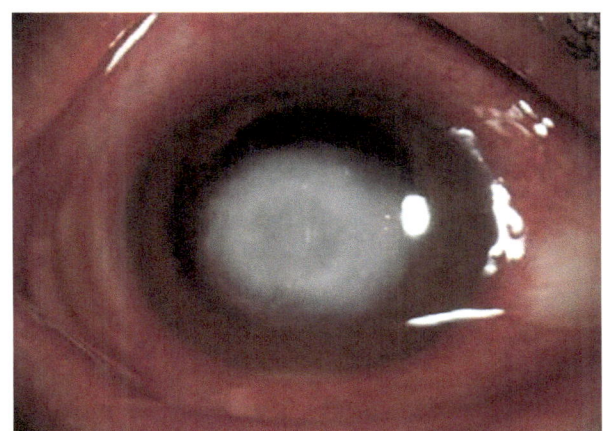

Fig. 4.23 *Acanthamoeba* keratitis at advanced stage, with stromal ulcer and dense stromal infiltration accompanied by hypopyon

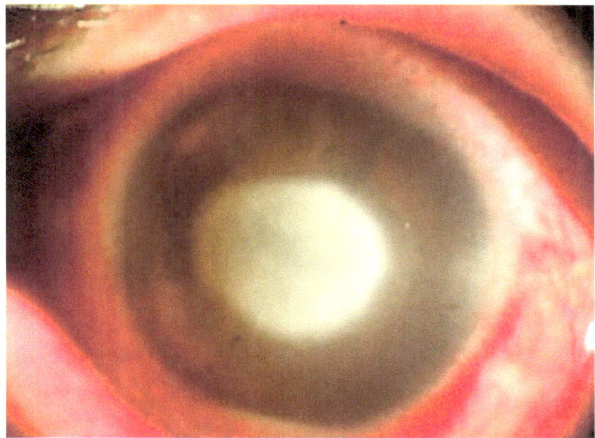

4.3.3   Late Stage

Patients at late stage usually have the deep stromal corneal ulcer of which the diameter is generally larger than 8 mm. It is often accompanied by obvious hypopyon or dense corneal stromal ring infiltration. *Ditch-shaped melting* at the periphery of the ulcer is deepened. Moreover, the thinning or even perforation is observed in the center of the corneal ulcer in some of patients, as shown in Figs. 4.24 and 4.25.

For a few of severe patients, the corneal inflammation or ulcer may involve corneoscleral *limbus* or even the sclera adjacent to the corneal limbus, resulting in corneal limbus inflammation (*limbitis*) with *neovascularization* or *anterior scleritis*. The corresponding manifestations include highly ciliary congestion and chemosis (Figs. 4.26, 4.27, 4.28, 4.29, 4.30, and 4.31). In addition, patients at late stage usually suffer from severe *ophthalmodynia*, *orbital pain*, or accompanying

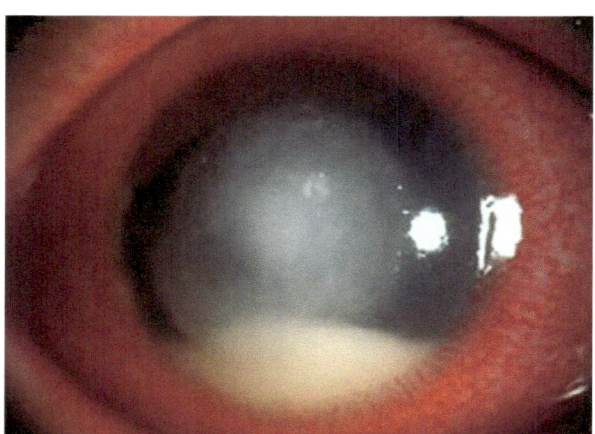

Fig. 4.24 *Acanthamoeba* keratitis at late stage, with lager and deep stromal ulcer accompanied by severe hypopyon

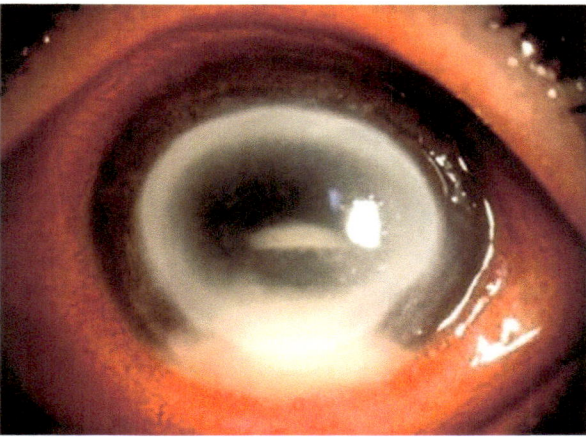

Fig. 4.25 *Acanthamoeba* keratitis at late stage, with lager and deep stromal ulcer with dense ring infiltration and severe hypopyon. The central area of the cornea is thinned

Fig. 4.26 *Acanthamoeba* keratitis at late stage, with ring infiltration and limbitis

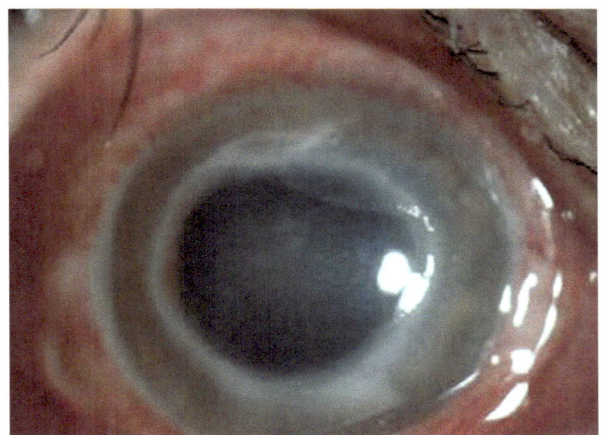

Fig. 4.27 *Acanthamoeba* keratitis at late stage with ring infiltration was limbitis

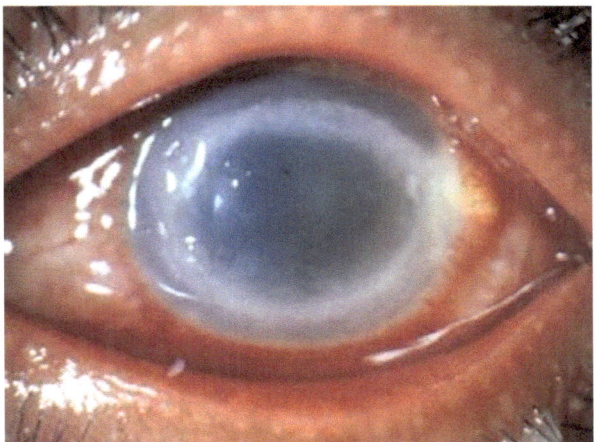

Fig. 4.28 *Acanthamoeba* keratitis at late stage, with dense ring infiltration and anterior scleritis. Neovascularization is observed at the peripheral cornea

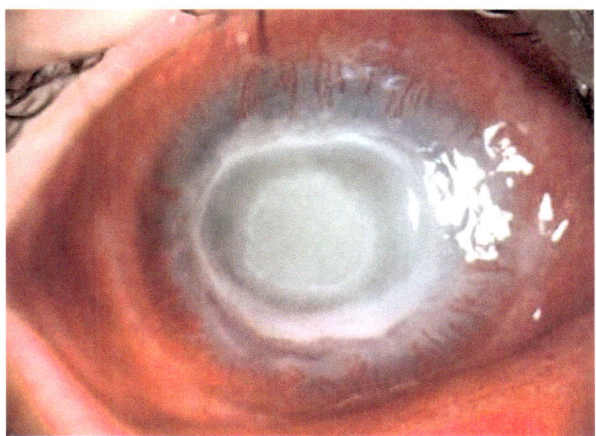

Fig. 4.29 *Acanthamoeba* keratitis at late stage, with dense ring infiltration and anterior scleritis

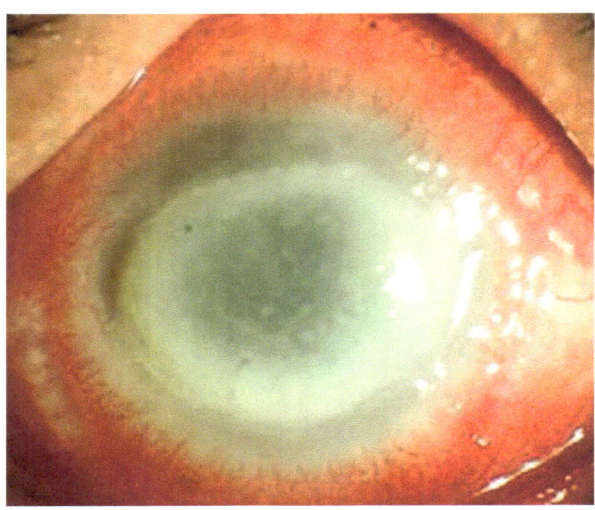

Fig. 4.30 At late stage, *Acanthamoeba* keratoscleritis with ditch-shaped melting in the corneal limbus. The central corneal area is thinned with hypopyon

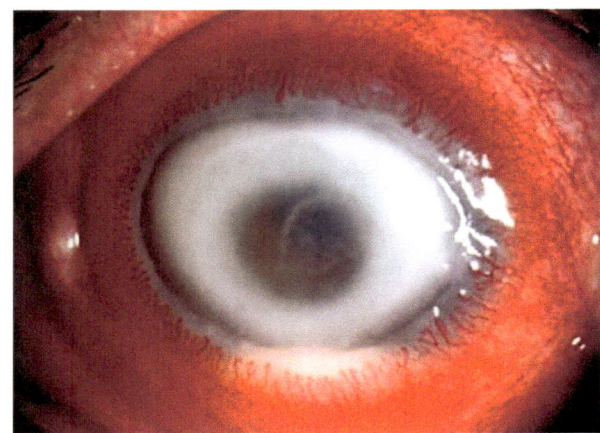

Fig. 4.31 At late stage, *Acanthamoeba* keratoscleritis with ditch-shaped melting involving the corneal limbus and anterior scleritis and subsequently glaucoma

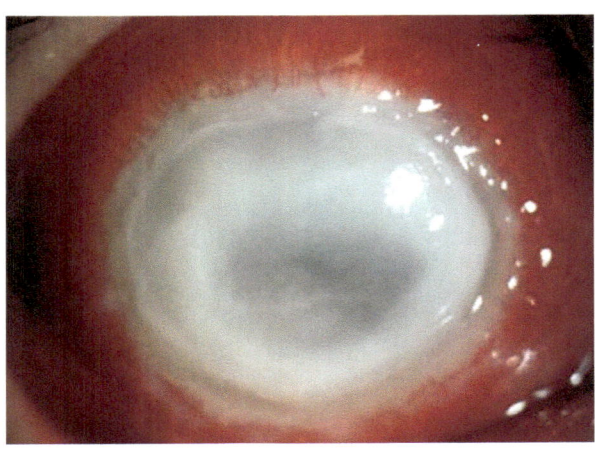

severe headache. Some patients may also have increased *intraocular pressure* and *secondary glaucoma*. As soon as the intraocular pressure continues to be increased, corneal ulcers become difficult to be cured. Furthermore, the tendency of corneal ulcer perforation may also increase.

4.4   Coinfection

Some of cases of *Acanthamoeba* keratitis may be coinfected with bacteria, fungi, viruses, and chlamydia. Fourteen cases of *Acanthamoeba* with coinfection had been collected from 1991 to 2014 in BIO. Out of these 14 cases, 9 cases were coinfected with bacteria, 4 cases of coinfection with fungus, and 1 case of coinfection with simple herpesvirus, as detailed in Table 4.6.

4.5   Complications

Patients with *Acanthamoeba* keratitis, especially those at advanced and late stages, are prone to have complications.

4.5.1   Anterior Uveitis

It is considered as an aseptic anterior chamber inflammatory reaction. Patients with mild symptoms show anterior chamber flash, planktonic cells, and keratic precipitates (KP). By contrast, hypopyon, pupil adhesion, and goniosynechia are observed for severe patients. The main cause of anterior uveitis is the stimulation of the corneal infectious inflammation. In addition, toxic reactions caused by long-term application of anti-amoeba drugs and the immunoreaction of the host to *Acanthamoeba* antigen also lead to the inflammations of anterior chamber.

Table 4.6 14 cases of *Acanthamoeba* keratitis coinfection with other microorganisms from 1991 to 2014 in BIO

Pathogens of mixed infection	No. of cases	Percentage (%)
Bacteria	9	64.3
Pseudomonas aeruginosa	3	
Staphylococcus epidermidis	4	
Staphylococcus aureus	1	
Klebsiella pneumoniae	1	
Fungi	4	28.6
Fusarium	1	
Aspergillus	1	
Undefined fungi	2	
Virus (herpes simplex virus)	1	7.1
Total	14	100.0

4.5.2   Intraocular Hypertension or Secondary Glaucoma

Patients at advanced stage and late stages and especially those with severe anterior chamber inflammatory reaction are prone to have intraocular hypertension or secondary glaucoma. During the clinical treatment, if intensified ophthalmodynia is complained and misty edema on the corneal epithelium is observed along with the stagnation of corneal ulcer healing process or aggravated ulcers with unknown reason, the occurrence of secondary intraocular hypertension and glaucoma should be taken into consideration. The intraocular pressure is around 30 mmHg for the majority of patients, which can be controlled by the application of topical antiglaucoma drugs and oral antiglaucoma drugs. However, these drugs might be not sufficient to the minority of patients who would require surgical treatment. The possible reasons of intraocular hypertension include the blockage of angles in anterior chamber by inflammatory substances, *atretopsia* resulted from anterior uveitis, and inflammation in the trabecular meshwork when the corneal limbitis involves the trabecular meshwork.

4.5.3   Anterior Scleritis

For a number of patients at late stage, corneal inflammation may lead to anterior scleritis. These patients often have severe ophthalmodynia accompanied by orbital pain and headache. Such serious pain usually influences patients' sleeping as well as the compliance of treatment. It is generally considered that immune reaction induced by *Acanthamoeba* antigens causes the scleritis. For these patients, topical nonsteroidal anti-inflammatory drugs and oral administration of analgesic anti-inflammatory drugs can control or relieve these symptoms.

4.5.4   Complicated Cataract

Patients of *Acanthamoeba* keratitis with the anterior uveitis, the pupil adhesion, long-term hypopyon, and repeated ulcer cautery with iodine tincture or corrosive are particularly prone to inducing complicated cataract.

In addition to the abovementioned complications, the majority of patients may have a series of accompanying reactions such as eyelid edema and congestion, chemosis, as well as blepharitis, which are related to the corneal inflammatory stimulation and the toxicity of anti-amoeba drugs.

References

1. Zhang C, Sun X. Diagnosis of bilateral *Acanthamoeba* keratitis related to orthokeratology with heidelberg retina tomograph III-RCM. Chin J Optom Ophthalmol. 2007;9(3):182–7.
2. Tian P, Sun X, Jin X. The combined infection of the cornea with *Acanthamoeba* and fungus. Chin J Ophthalmol. 2000;36(4):298.
3. Jin X, Luo S, Zhang W. Diagnosis and prevention of *Acanthamoeba* keratitis. Ophthalmol CHN. 1992;1(2):67–71.
4. Wilhelmus KR, Jones DB, Matoba AY, et al. Bilateral *Acanthamoeba* keratitis. Am J Ophthalmol. 2008;145(2):193–7.
5. Tu EY, Joslin CE, Sugar J, et al. Prognostic factors affecting visual outcome in *Acanthamoeba* keratitis. Ophthalmology. 2008;115(11):1998–2003.
6. Gao M, Zhang Y, Li R, et al. *Acanthamoeba* keratitis: clinical characteristics and management. Chin J Ocul Trauma Occup Eye Dis. 2006;28(5):331–4.
7. Sun X, Jin X. *Acanthamoeba* keratitis. Ophthalmol CHN. 2002;11(1):4–6.
8. Sun X, Zhang Y, Li R, et al. *Acanthamoeba* keratitis: clinical characteristics and management. Ophthalmology. 2006;113(3):412–6.
9. Zhang C, Deng S, Wang Z, et al. Clinical synthetic diagnosis and management of *Acanthamoeba* keratitis. Ophthalmol CHN. 2008;17(2):104–8.

Diagnosis and Differential Diagnosis

5

5.1 Diagnosis of *Acanthamoeba* Keratitis

5.1.1 Clinical Diagnosis

The clinical diagnosis of *Acanthamoeba* keratitis is mainly based on the following aspects:

1. Risk factors: common risk factors include *agricultural trauma*, corneal contact lenses wear, splashing of foreign matters or small insects, etc.
2. *Onset time*: the disease gradually progresses in 3–7 days after being affected by one or more risk factors.
3. Characteristics of the *corneal signs* (Fig. 5.1a–d):
   (a) Typical corneal ring infiltration
   (b) Ditch-shaped melting at the edge of corneal ulcer
   (c) Crude salt-like granular dense infiltration
   (d) Radial keratoneuritis

However, at the early stage of *Acanthamoeba* keratitis, the corneal signs are often not typical. Therefore, it is rather difficult to make clinical diagnosis just based on early corneal signs of keratitis.

5.1.2 Etiological Diagnosis

Etiological diagnosis can be done by laboratory examinations (the examination methods in detail are seen in Chap. 6). The common *laboratory examinations* include as follows:

1. Smear cytological examinations of corneal scraping
   (a) Wet mount method, i.e., direct observation is carried out after smear

© Springer Nature Singapore Pte Ltd.
& People's Medical Publishing House, PR of China 2018
X. Sun, *Acanthamoeba Keratitis*, https://doi.org/10.1007/978-981-10-5212-5_5

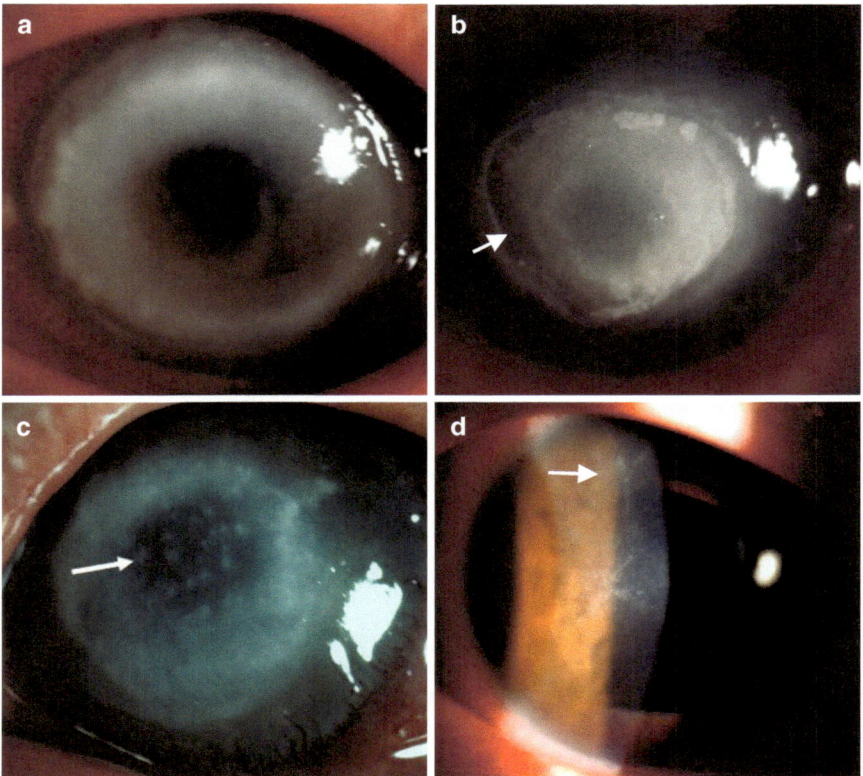

Fig. 5.1 (**a–d**) Typical corneal signs of *Acanthamoeba* keratitis. (**a**) Ring infiltration. (**b**) Ditch-shaped melting (shown by white arrow). (**c**) Crude salt-like granular infiltration (shown by white arrow). (**d**) Radial keratoneuritis (shown by white arrow)

(b) Staining method, i.e., the observation is carried out after the staining of the smear (e.g., Giemsa staining)

The cytological examination of *scraping* on necrotic tissue of the corneal ulcer area is generally considered as the fastest, simple, and convenient laboratory method for etiological diagnosis of *Acanthamoeba* keratitis. Once the proficiency in this method is obtained, it shows the higher detection rate of pathogens than other methods used in clinical laboratory. More specifically, the detection of typical cysts and trophozoites obtained from scraping smear can be utilized as a guide for *etiological diagnosis*.

With scraping cytology examination, stained smears show higher *detection rate* of pathogens and more accuracy rate than wet mount method. Amoebic cyst with varying forms is the most commonly detected pathogen in scrape cytology, including cysts at mature stage with complete structure, cysts at *the cyst prophase* that are being transformed from trophozoites, and *empty cysts* without cell contents which have not vitality. Any one of cysts forms abovementioned is significantly important for the etiological diagnosis. By contrast, the opportunity of detecting *Acanthamoeba* trophozoite in the corneal smear is relatively not common [1].

2. Cultivation of amoeba

   The culture method is the golden standard for *Acanthamoeba* etiological diagnosis. However, the cultivation of amoeba requires special non-nutrition culture medium and, simultaneously, the addition of *E. coli*. Moreover it normally takes 10–12 days to observe the growth of *Acanthamoeba* trophozoite. Hence, it is difficult to make *rapid etiological diagnosis* depending on culture method.

3. Examination by in vivo corneal laser scanning confocal microscope

   The corneal confocal microscopy can be applied to observe the typical amoebic cyst in vivo in the corneal tissues of patients and make etiological diagnosis according to the image of typical cysts usually or trophozoite sometime. However, the observation with the corneal confocal microscope might be affected by various aspects, including the change of the corneal tissue transparency (e.g., by inflammatory infiltration and the severe corneal edema) and the change of cellular constituent in the corneal tissues (e.g., activated corneal stromal cells and infiltration of a variety of inflammatory cells) and so on. As a consequence, the image of *Acanthamoeba* cyst might be not typical at some of time. Thus, the possibility of *Acanthamoeba* keratitis cannot be entirely excluded even if no typical cyst is observed in clinical examination with the corneal confocal microscopy. Accordingly, the results obtained by the corneal confocal microscopy should be carefully analyzed by combining microbiological tests, clinical manifestations, risk factors, and medical history.

   For patients that are highly suspected suffering from *Acanthamoeba* keratitis, the examination by in vivo the corneal laser scanning confocal microscope should be repeated, which is found beneficial for the confirmation of etiological and differential diagnosis. When the diagnosis is set up, in vivo the corneal laser scanning confocal microscope could be helpful for evaluating the effect of the therapy during the management of infection [2–4].

   The single-wavelength laser beam emitted from the laser light source system is focalized, passes through the left fissure hole of the scanning fissure system, and enters the optical lens system. The beam gets through left side of the lens system and is focalized on a certain focal plane which is located inside the corneal tissue. The light beam reflected from the focal plane inside the corneal tissue is focalized by passing through the right side of the optical lens system and then gets through the right fissure hole of the scanning fissure system. Finally, the data of this beam is assembled by a digital optical collector and transported to the computer system for analysis and processing. Subsequently, the image of the corneal focal plane can be displayed. The theoretical *resolution* of in vivo corneal *laser scanning confocal microscope* is 1 micrometer (μm), and the average *magnification* is 800.

   Typical *Acanthamoeba* cysts can be observed with the in vivo corneal laser scanning confocal microscope. Sometimes, trophozoites can also be found in the corneal tissues. According to different stages of keratitis, the *Acanthamoeba* cysts display various images of typical forms, which mainly include *double-walled cyst*, empty cyst, *solid cyst*, *star-like cyst*, and *cyst surrounded by a dark ring*. The diameter of the cysts is generally between 10 and 15 μm [5]. *Acanthamoeba* trophozoites have irregular shapes and show medium density of reflection in the confocal microscope images. In the center of the trophozoites, the nucleus is observed as a circular dark area, the center of which is dense and highly reflective. The diameter of the trophozoites is approximately 25 μm (Figs. 5.2, 5.3, 5.4, 5.5, 5.6, and 5.7).

Fig. 5.2 A circular *Acanthamoeba* cyst with the diameter of around 15 μm (shown by the white arrow). Both the wall of cyst and the contents inside the cyst show high reflective image

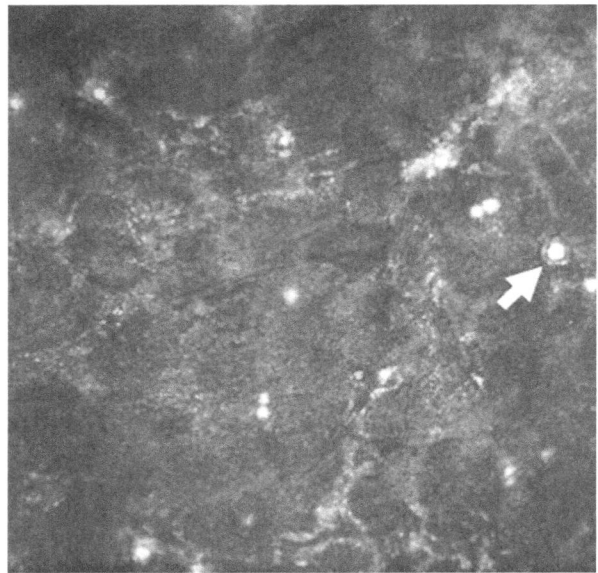

Fig. 5.3 An empty *Acanthamoeba* cyst (shown by the white arrow). Low reflective image can be observed inside the cyst

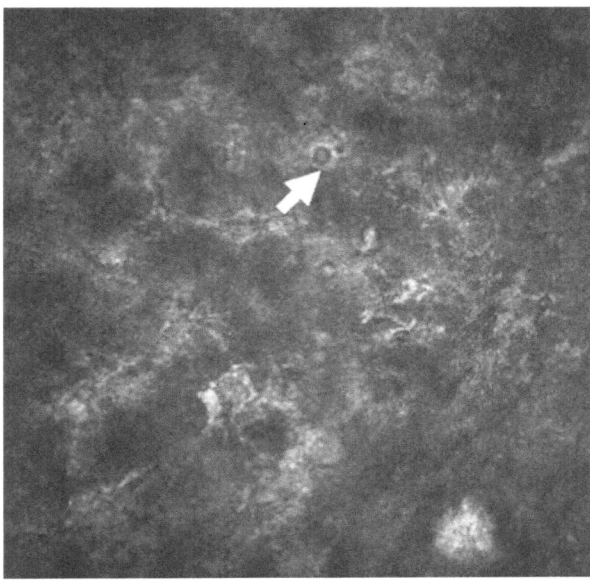

Fig. 5.4 The *Acanthamoeba* cysts display circular and highly reflective (shown by the white arrow)

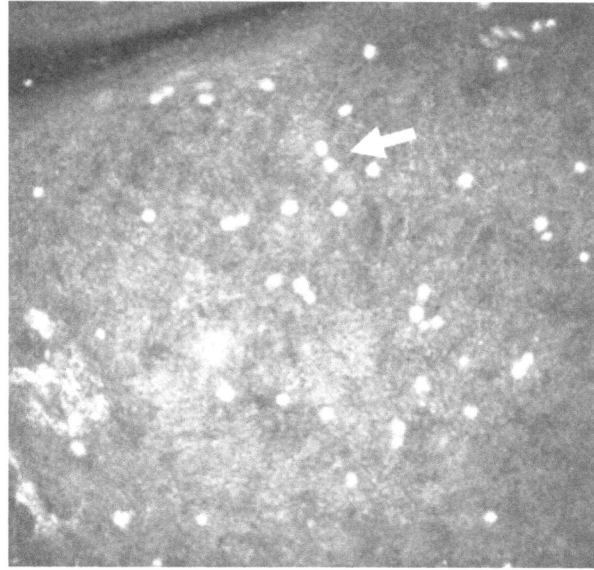

Fig. 5.5 The *Acanthamoeba* cysts display circular and highly reflective. The wall of the cysts shows a polygonal in shape. The cysts are clustered (shown by the white arrow), and the diameter of the cyst is about 10 μm

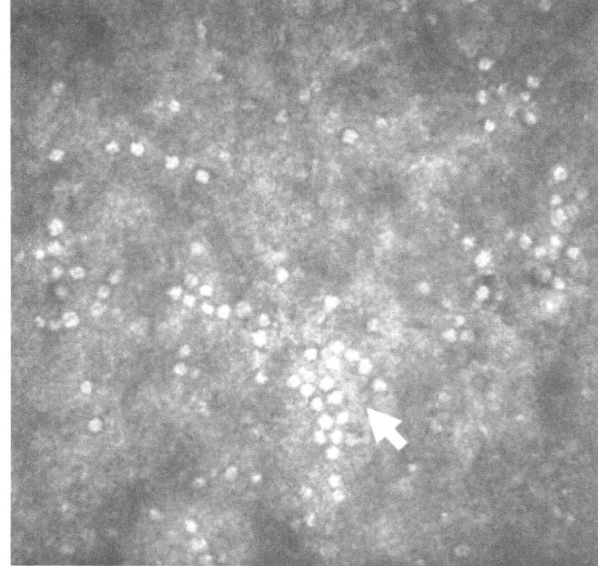

   In the observation with the corneal confocal laser scanning microscope, *Acanthamoeba* cysts may display *scattered, clustered,* or *string-like arrangements* (Figs. 5.8 and 5.9). When *Acanthamoeba* cysts in the cornea tissues present clustered or string-like arrangement, it is often an indication that the patients are in more severe condition and anti-amoeba drugs may have poor effects to patients. Surgical managements usually are needed immediately for these patients.

Fig. 5.6 A lot of
Acanthamoeba cysts in the
corneal stoma (shown by
the black arrow)

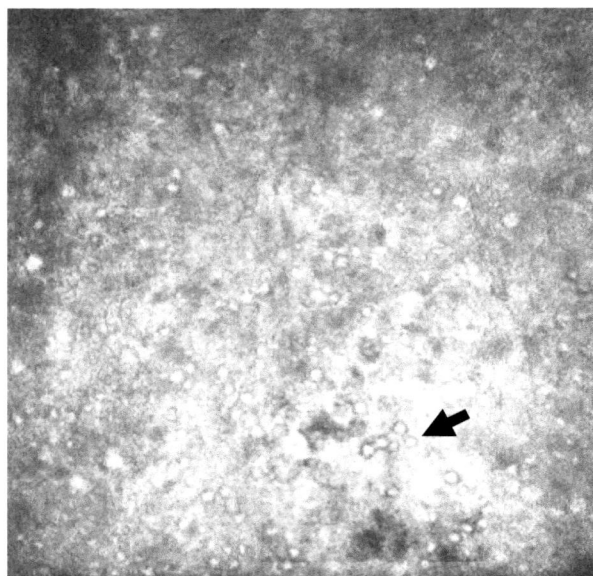

Fig. 5.7 The
Acanthamoeba trophozoite
in the corneal stoma
(shown by the black arrow)

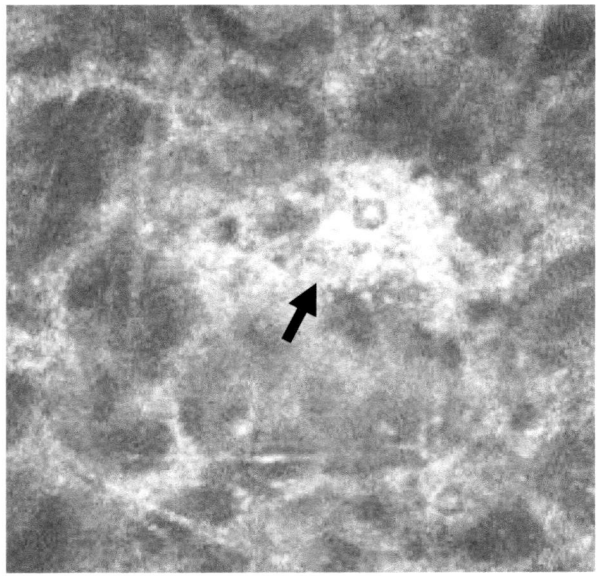

   The examination with the corneal confocal laser scanning microscope can
indicate the *depth* of the cornea tissue in which *Acanthamoeba* cysts are involved
(Figs. 5.10 and 5.11). According to the repeated observations of such depths during therapy of the patients, the degree of severity of the disease and the effect to
therapy of anti-amoeba drugs can be assessed.

Fig. 5.8 The
Acanthamoeba cysts show
scattered arrangement

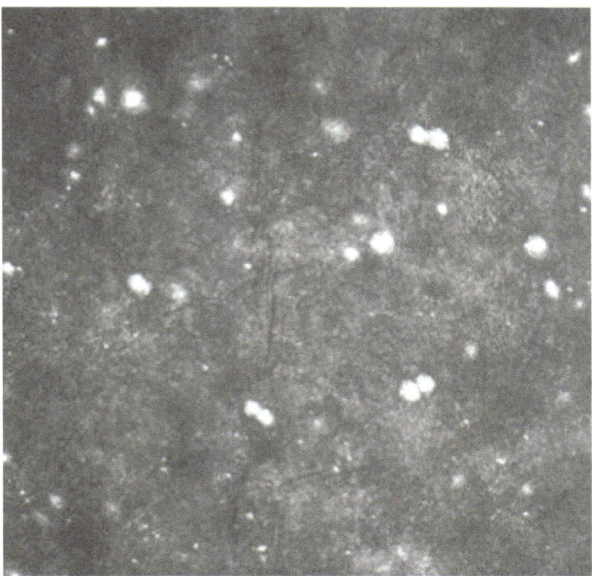

Fig. 5.9 The
Acanthamoeba cysts show
clustered (red arrow) and
string-like arrangements
(white arrow)

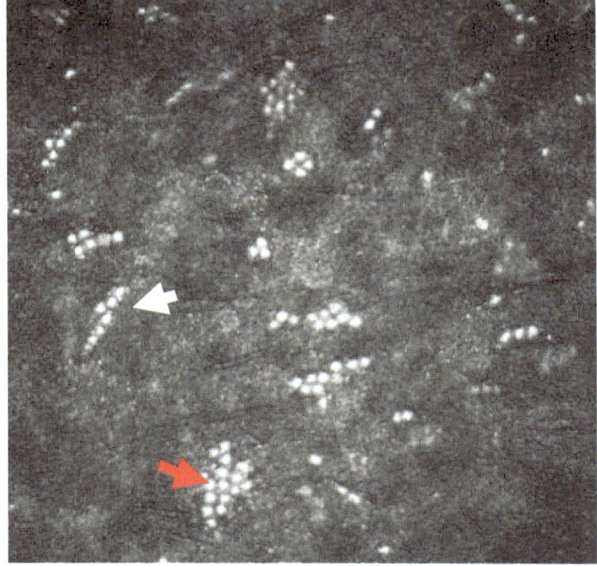

   During the observation with the corneal confocal microscope, *air bubbles*
may be remained in the contact interface between the cornea surface and the
inner surface of the plastic lens cap, which is more frequently observed in
patients who have the deep corneal ulcers (Figs. 5.12 and 5.13). Under the corneal confocal microscope, air bubbles that are lager dot-like structures with high

Fig. 5.10 Multiple cysts
are observed at the depth
of 163 μm in the corneal
stroma

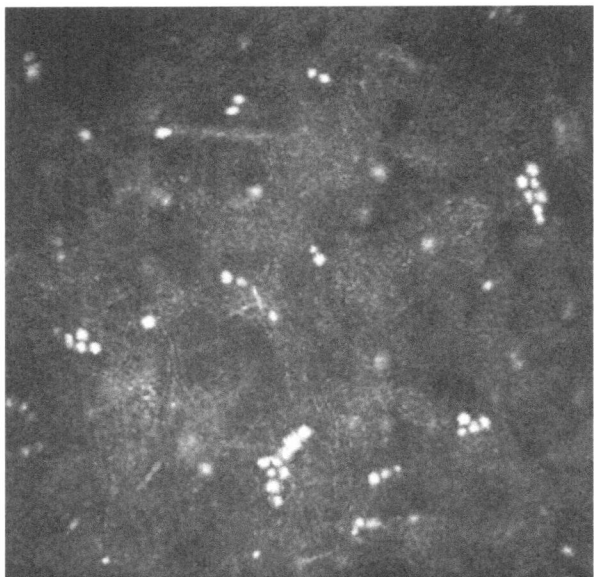

Fig. 5.11 A large number
of cysts are found at the
depth of 283 μm in the
corneal stroma

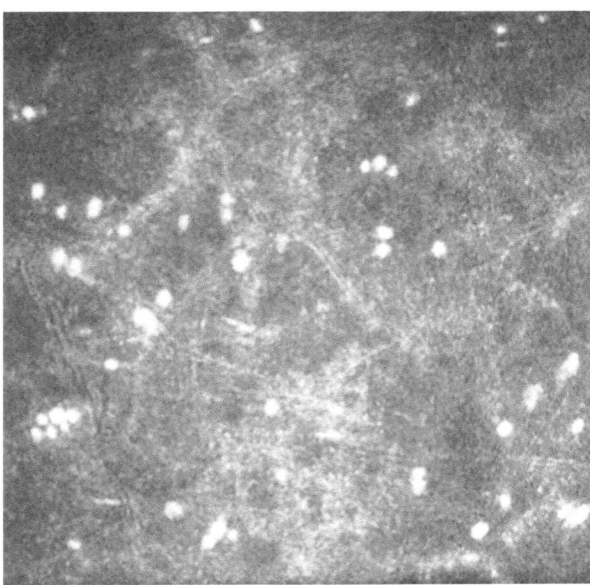

density of reflection and varying diameters can be observed. The images of air
bubbles are prone to be confused with *Acanthamoeba* cysts. In general, the air
bubbles are located on the surface of the cornea. The diameters of air bubbles are
bigger than that of cysts and vary significantly. The air bubbles display *a high*

Fig. 5.12 Bubbles are found between plastic lens cap of confocal microscope and the corneal surface, (shown by the white arrow). The bubbles have high reflective in the center with a diameter ranging from 30 to 50 μm

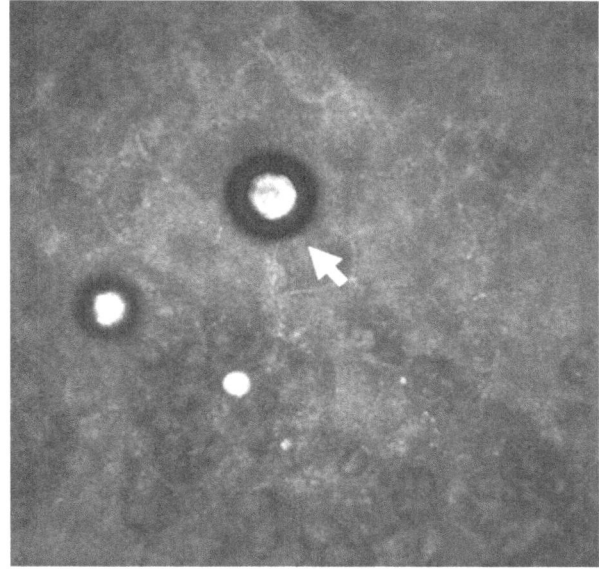

Fig. 5.13 Bubbles are observed between plastic lens cap of the confocal microscope and corneal surface (shown by the white arrow)

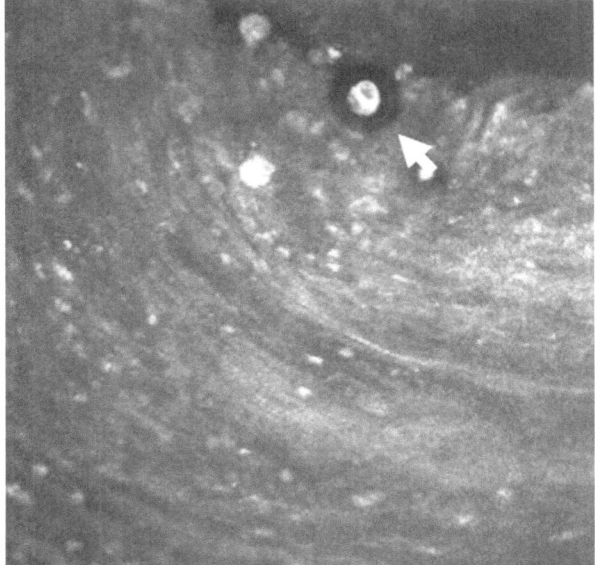

reflection in the center, and lower reflection is observed in ring area around the center. When slightly pressing the plastic lens cap during the examination, the position of the air bubbles is shifted immediately or the air bubbles can be disappeared, which is very helpful for *identification*.

4. Polymerase chain reaction (PCR)

   The application of polymerase chain reaction (PCR) amplification on partial sequence containing DF3 of *Acanthamoeba 18S rDNA* through specific primers JDP1-JDP2 is the most commonly used method for the diagnosis of *Acanthamoeba*. Although the cultivation of *Acanthamoeba* is the golden standard for etiological diagnosis of *Acanthamoeba* keratitis, a relatively small number of pathogens often result in false-negative results, and the culture will take several days to observe the results. Many studies have confirmed that PCR technique is very useful in the *rapid diagnosis* of *Acanthamoeba*, which generally takes several hours for reporting the results. It has been reported that one to ten trophozoites could be detected by PCR [6, 7].

5.2   Differential Diagnosis of *Acanthamoeba* Keratitis

When typical corneal ring infiltration, ditch-shaped melting at the edge of corneal ulcer, crude salt-like granular dense infiltration, and radial keratoneuritis are presented, the clinical diagnosis of *Acanthamoeba* keratitis is relatively not difficult to be considered. However, when the corneal infection is at the early stage or the corneal signs of *Acanthamoeba* keratitis are atypical, it is usually misdiagnosed as the viral keratitis or fungal keratitis. Hence, comprehensive analysis and careful assessment based on clinical manifestations are required. Furthermore, the diagnostic value of laboratory examination is particularly essential.

5.2.1   Key Points for Differential Diagnosis of *Acanthamoeba* Keratitis from Viral Keratitis

1. *Risk factors*. The majority of patients with viral keratitis have risk factors including fever, fatigue, emotional stress, and decreased immunity. By contrast, most of the patients with *Acanthamoeba* keratitis usually have trauma or history of the corneal contact lens wear, which is an essential point in the clinical differential diagnosis to be considered firstly.
2. *Medical history*. Viral keratitis patients often have a history of *recurrent attacks* of the keratitis. If a patient used to have a history of recurrent viral keratitis, it is helpful for the differential diagnosis by combining risk factors. Generally speaking, only few patients with *Acanthamoeba* keratitis report a history of recurrent keratitis. However, it should be noted in clinical practice that, in some of *Acanthamoeba* keratitis patients at early stage which have been misdiagnosed as viral keratitis, their corneal infection might be relieved after the combined application of antiviral drugs and glucocorticoids temporarily. Nonetheless, the condition significantly worsened after long-term application of glucocorticoids. In clinical practice, such situation should be distinguished from the recurrence of viral keratitis.

3. *Corneal signs*. Viral epithelial infected keratitis usually presents *dendritic ulcer*, geographic ulcer, and marginal keratitis with apparently positive staining with fluorescein. The typical dendritic ulcer has the features of a branching, linear lesion with terminal bulbs, and swollen epithelial borders. At the early stage of *Acanthamoeba* keratitis, *pseudodendrites* is observed in the corneal epithelium layer. The epithelium in pseudodendrites region is ridged with the mild punctate or clustered corneal fluorescein staining. But no swollen epithelial borders are observed.
4. Efficacy of treatment with antiviral drugs. Viral epithelial infected keratitis at early stage, such as dendritic ulcer, geographic ulcer, and marginal keratitis, will be apparently improved after the treatment of antiviral drugs for 1–2 weeks. By contrast, no significant effect with therapy of antiviral drugs is observed for *Acanthamoeba* keratitis patients. As for *Acanthamoeba* keratitis patients at early stage, the application of anti-amoeba drugs may enable releasing their symptoms and signs significantly.
5. Examination by corneal confocal microscopy. In the examination with the corneal confocal microscopy, small and circular inflammatory cell images usually can be found in the corneal epithelium layer or in the corneal stroma for viral keratitis patients. On the contrary, for *Acanthamoeba* keratitis patients at early stage, only few inflammatory cells are found in corneal tissues. Typical images of *Acanthamoeba* cysts usually can be observed.

5.2.2 Key Points of Differential Diagnosis of *Acanthamoeba* Keratitis from Fungal Keratitis

1. *Risk factors*. Risk factors of fungal keratitis often are similar to those of *Acanthamoeba* keratitis. Therefore, it is difficult to make differential diagnosis just based on the types of risk factors.
2. *Medical history*. Fungal keratitis displays similar *onset process* with *Acanthamoeba* keratitis, i.e., patients generally show gradual onset of disease within 3–7 days after the exposure to risk factors. However, after the onset of fungal keratitis, yellow-white purulent infiltration or ulcer is observed for most of patients. By contrast, *Acanthamoeba* keratitis often exhibits epithelial punctuate keratopathy, pseudodendrites, or gray-white dense and non-purulent corneal infiltration. Furthermore, for fungal keratitis, inflammation reaction of anterior chamber or hypopyon is apparent. As for *Acanthamoeba* keratitis at early stage, only mild or no inflammation reaction in the anterior chamber is observed.
3. *Corneal signs*. In addition to the corneal purulent infiltration and ulcer, a characteristic corneal signs of fungal keratitis are *feathery margins* and *elevated edges* of the ulcer with rough texture and satellite lesions. These changes except for satellite lesions are barely observed in *Acanthamoeba* keratitis patients. Since *satellite lesions* can be observed in both fungal and *Acanthamoeba* keratitis, it cannot be used as an evidence for differential diagnosis.

4. Corneal smear cytology examination is the fast and effective method for differentiating fungal or *Acanthamoeba* corneal infections. If typical *fungal hyphae* are detected in the corneal smears, fungal keratitis can be diagnosed. But at some of time, repeat corneal smear cytology examinations will be needed for etiology diagnosis.
5. Corneal laser scanning confocal microscopy also is the fast and effective method for distinguishing in vivo fungal or *Acanthamoeba* corneal infections. If images of typical hyphae or *Acanthamoeba* cysts are observed, etiology diagnosis will be set up.

5.2.3   Key Points of Differential Diagnosis of *Acanthamoeba* Keratitis from Bacterial Keratitis

1. *Risk factors.* The risk factors of bacterial and *Acanthamoeba* keratitis are analogous. Therefore, it is impossible to differentiate from one to another only on the basis of risk factors.
2. *Medical history.* Bacterial keratitis, especially the acute keratitis caused by *pyogenic bacteria*, often shows *rapid onset*, i.e., within 1–3 days after the exposure of risk factors. The corneal ulcer or corneal *purulent infiltration* is rapidly formed and progressed, usually accompanied by *severe hypopyon* in the anterior chamber, which is important point for differentiating bacterial keratitis from *Acanthamoeba* keratitis because *Acanthamoeba* keratitis generally presents the features of subacute or chronic onset and gradual progression.
3. The *corneal signs.* Bacterial keratitis displays yellow-white purulent infiltration or the corneal ulcer. A large amount of purulent *necrotic tissues* or *discharges* are often found on the surface of the corneal ulcer. In addition, satellite lesion is rather rare in bacterial keratitis patients. The application of broad-spectrum antibiotics in *intensified therapy* generally shows obvious efficacy for bacterial corneal ulcer. However, antibiotics commonly used are not effective for *Acanthamoeba* keratitis.
4. The corneal smear cytology examination and bacterial culture. Varying amounts of bacteria can be observed in the corneal smear cytology examination for bacterial keratitis patients, indicating the possibility of bacterial infection. The bacterial culture is the golden standard for etiological diagnosis of bacterial keratitis, and it can provide results of the antibiotics sensitivity which is helpful to guide the physicians to select correct medications. The bacterial culture generally will take 2–3 days to get test reports from laboratory.

References

1. Wang ZQ, Li R, Zhang C, et al. Morphological characteristics in corneal smear of acanthamoeba keratitis. Zhonghua Yan Ke Za Zhi. 2010;46(5):432–6. Chinese.
2. Hang L, Wang L, Liuhe Z, et al. Clinical diagnosis of Acanthamoeba keratitis with confocal microscopy. Ophthalmol CHN. 2003;12(6):336–8.
3. Sun X, Pang G, Wang Z. Diagnosis of Acanthamoeba keratitis with in vivo confocal microscopy. Chin J Ophthalmol. 1999;35(5):400.
4. Chen Z, Xuguang S. Diagnosis of bilateral Acanthamoeba keratitis related to orthokeratology with Heidelberg retina yomograph III-RCM. Chin J Optom Ophthalmol. 2007;9(3):182–7.
5. Zhang C, Deng S, Wang Z, et al. Diagnosis evaluation of Acanthamoeba keratitis with Heidelberg retina tomograph III-RCM. Chin Ophthalmic Res. 2007;25(10):772–4.
6. Yan Z, Xuguang S. Genotype and identification of Acanthamoeba. Sect Ophthalmol Foreign Med Sci. 2002;26(4):214–7.
7. Jiang C, Liang Q, Sun X. Genotyping of Acanthamoeba isolated from keratitis and clinical signification. Int Rev Ophthalmol. 2011;35(4):232–6.

Laboratory Examination

With the increasing cases of *Acanthamoeba* keratitis, more clinical requirements are needed for laboratory tests for etiology diagnosis. The main roles of laboratory examination for *Acanthamoeba* include: (1) the *etiological diagnosis* of pathogen, (2) the *evaluating efficacy* of therapy, and (3) the *estimation of prognosis* of the diseases. At present, the laboratory examination methods commonly used for the ocular infection of *Acanthamoeba* mainly are divided into two categories, i.e., the conventional examination method and special examination method.

The *conventional examination* methods generally do not require special equipment and are easy for application in clinical ocular microbiological laboratory. These methods mainly consist of: (1) scraping cytology examination (Giemsa stain and direct wet mount), (2) culture of *Acanthamoeba*, (3) in vitro anti-amoeba drug susceptibility test, (4) histopathological examination, and (5) flagellum test.

By contrast, the *special examination* methods require more special devices or special reagents, which mainly contain: (1) special staining, (2) electronic microscopy observation, and (3) molecular biology test.

6.1   Method of the Cornea *Sample Collection*

The quality of a laboratory's definitive diagnosis of pathogens is depended on proper collection and expeditious handling of specimens, using appropriate stains for smear and culture media or other procedures. In order to ensure the reliability and validity of the examination results, the correct collection of the corneal specimen is the first step of the critical procedures of laboratory techniques. The *qualified specimen* should be extracted from appropriate location and depth of the corneal lesions, and contain sufficient sample amount for the smear, culture, or other tests. Moreover, the specimen should be clearly labeled and correctly handled. Most importantly, any of the specimens collected from the patients should be *rapidly delivered* to the laboratory for examination.

© Springer Nature Singapore Pte Ltd.
& People's Medical Publishing House, PR of China 2018
X. Sun, *Acanthamoeba Keratitis*, https://doi.org/10.1007/978-981-10-5212-5_6

6.1.1   Sample Collection for the Cornea Smear Cytology Examination

The sample collection method includes three steps:

Step 1: The *glass slide* should be cleaned by medical ethanol 75% and then steril-ized using alcohol lamp flame. In addition, the range of smeared sample location on the surface of glass slide for observation and sample number should be *labeled* by marker pen. Moreover, the *Kimura platinum spatula* for sample collection also has to be sterilized with alcohol lamp flame.

Step 2: After the cornea is anesthetized with a *topical anesthetic*, a lid speculum is placed to expose the surface of the cornea lesions. The corneal ulcer is scraped using Kimura spatula and the advancing edge of the corneal ulcer or the necrotic side is debrided in addition to the base of the ulcer. If necessary, the sample col-lection may be operated under slit lamp bio-microscope or surgical operation microscope in order to avoid the damage of the normal corneal tissues and the prevention of the perforation or the hemorrhage.

Step 3: The samples obtained for the cornea are smeared directly onto two or three clean glass slides in *monolayer* as far as possible. The smeared samples on the glass slides are fixed with methanol 95% and after air-dry for 5 min the glass slides are submitted to the laboratory for observation immediately.

6.1.2   Sample Collection for the Culture of *Acanthamoeba*

After the cornea is anesthetized with a topical anesthetic, a lid speculum is placed to expose the surface of the cornea lesions. The corneal ulcer is scraped using Kimura spatula and the advancing edge or the necrotic side is debrided in addition to the base of the ulcer. Then the scraped or *debrided* samples of the corneal lesions are collected using sterilized *transport swabs* that should be placed on the corneal ulcer area for at least 5 s in order to obtain more amount of material from the ulcer. Then transport swabs are submitted to the laboratory for culture of *Acanthamoeba* as soon as possible.

6.2   Conventional Methods of Examination

6.2.1   *Smear Cytological Examination* of the Corneal Scraping

The corneal scraping smear cytological examination is a simple and rapid method for etiology diagnosis conventionally used in clinical practice and generally can identify the types of the pathogens in several hours. The positive rate of the corneal scraping smear cytological examination for *Acanthamoeba* is 82.4% [1]. Trophozoites, mature cysts, pre-cysts, and empty cysts of *Acanthamoeba* can be observed in smear exami-nation, and with the finding any one of these forms of *Acanthamoeba,* etiological diagnosis of *Acanthamoeba keratitis* could be set up [2–8].

Giemsa Stain Method

Giemsa stain is the cytologic stain most commonly used for ophthalmic specimens. Because of its staining properties, Giemsa stain is considered as a beneficial method in the diagnoses of parasitic infection.

1. Sample collection: The sample collection and preparation is carried out according to the sample collection method of smear of the corneal scraping mentioned above.
2. *Fixation*: Fix slide in methanol 95% for 5 min, allowing the slide to air-dry.
3. *Staining*: Giemsa stock solution is diluted to Giemsa working solution with a ratio of 1:10 by using phosphate buffer with pH 7.0 and 1/15 mol/L or distilled water. The working solution (5–6 drops) is placed on the glass slide. The staining lasts 15–20 min in the incubator at 37 °C. Then the working solution is rinsed off carefully using phosphate buffer or distilled water and the slide is allowed to air-dry. Under a brightfield light microscope, the slide is observed.

   The preparation of Giemsa solution

   (a) The preparation of Giemsa stock solution: stock solution contains Giemsa powder (0.5 g), neutral glycerol (33 mL), and methanol (33 mL), which is preserved at 4 °C usually.
   (b) the preparation of working solution: by diluting the Giemsa stock solution using phosphate buffer with pH 7.0 and 1/15 mol/L or distilled water with a ratio of 1:10, which should be freshly prepared before use.

4. Observation under the light microscope: The *Acanthamoeba trophozoite* is oval, quasi-circular, oblong, or irregular in shape with a diameter of 15–45 μm. Spines and pseudopodia can be observed. The cell nucleus is generally located in the central area of the cell and stained in the color of dark blue. A transparent zone can be found around the nucleus with a dense nucleolus in the center of the nucleus. Reticular, vacuoles and blue or purple particles can be seen in the cytoplasm (Figs. 6.1, 6.2, 6.3, and 6.4). Since *Acanthamoeba* trophozoites are fragile

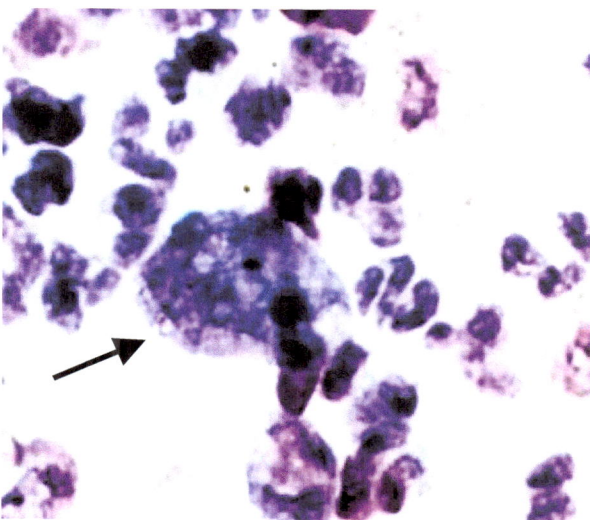

Fig. 6.1 *Acanthamoeba* trophozoite (shown by arrow) is oval in shape and contains vacuoles in the plasma (Giemsa stain, ×1000)

Fig. 6.2 *Acanthamoeba* trophozoite (shown by arrow) is oval in shape. There are a lot of porous and reticular structures in the cytoplasm (Giemsa stain, ×1000)

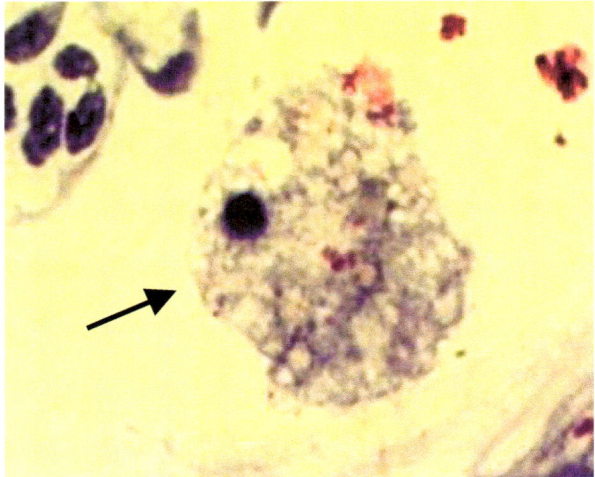

Fig. 6.3 *Acanthamoeba* trophozoite (shown by arrow) is oval in shape and the vacuoles can be observed in the plasma (Giemsa stain, ×1000)

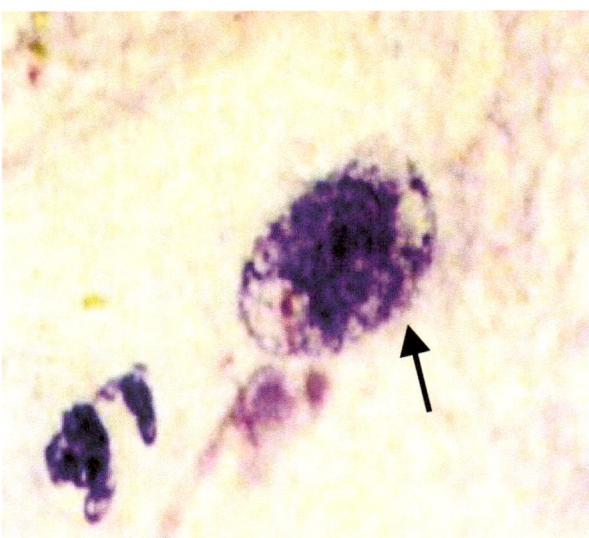

and may be easily broken during smearing and staining procedures, it is not common to observe trophozoites in the smear examination of the corneal scraping.

Under the light microscope, cyst is the most commonly structure observed in smear examination of the corneal scraping. The cyst at mature stage is round, or polygonal in shape with a diameter of between 10 and 20 μm and the typical double-wall structure of cyst usually is found. The *outer* wall of the cyst (i.e., *ectocyst*) is often folded, lace-like or wrinkled whereas the *inner* wall of the cyst (i.e., *endocyst*) is smooth and polygonal, circular, star-like or triangular in shape. Both ectocyst and endocyst are stained in the color of blue with Giemsa stain. There is a *transparent gap* between these two layers which is generally not

Fig. 6.4 *Acanthamoeba* trophozoite (shown by arrow) that begins to transform to pre-cyst, but the double-wall of cyst is not yet fully formed (Giemsa stain, ×1000)

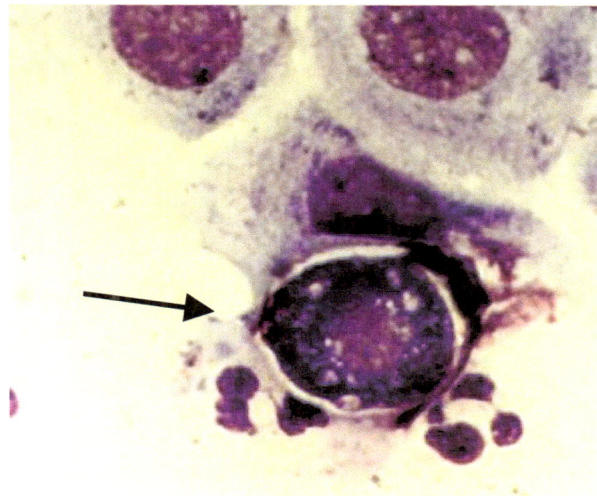

Fig. 6.5 A cyst is spherical in shape with a double-wall. Dense nucleus and nucleolus (shown by white arrow. Giemsa stain, ×1000)

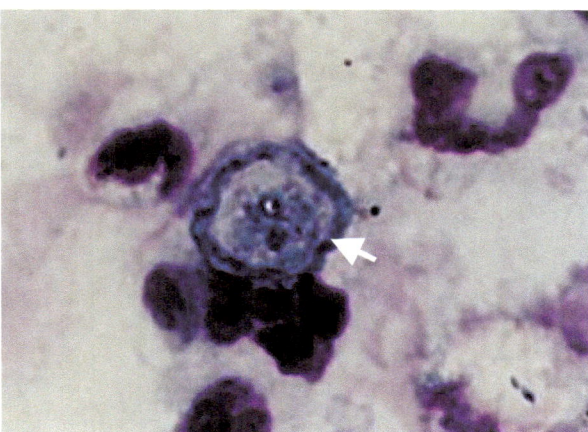

stained. The cytoplasm of the cyst is very dense with many granules in the color of dark blue, light blue, or light pink according to the time of staining and the cell nucleus is usually in the color of dark blue with a nucleolus that is similar to that of trophozoite (Figs. 6.5 and 6.6).

Pre-cyst (the cyst prophase) is an amebic form that is transforming from trophozoite to mature cyst and the size of pre-cyst is slightly larger than that of mature cyst. The double-wall of pre-cyst is not completely formed or only formed with a single-layer wall and the latter is not stained by Giemsa stain (Figs. 6.7 and 6.8). In addition, the *cytoplasmic granules* inside the cell are relatively coarse and large in color of blue-purple without vacuoles. Furthermore, an obvious nucleus in color of dark blue can be observed in pre-cyst.

Fig. 6.6 A cyst is
pentagonal in shape with a
thin double-wall (Giemsa
stain, ×1000)

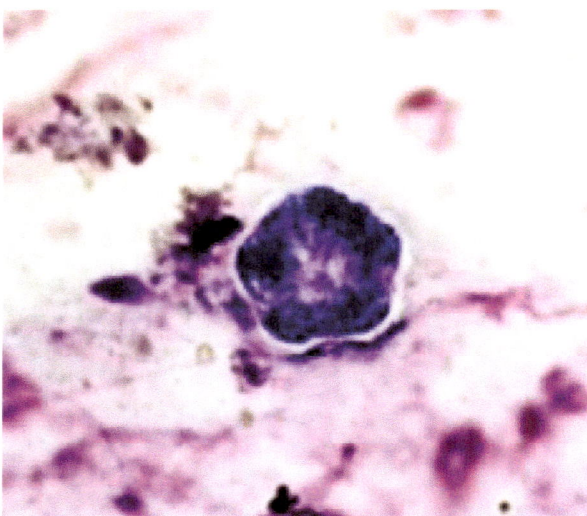

Fig. 6.7 Pre-cyst (shown
by yellow arrows) with a
smooth, single-layer wall.
There are dense granules in
the cytoplasm with an
obvious nucleus and a
nucleolus (Giemsa stain,
×1000)

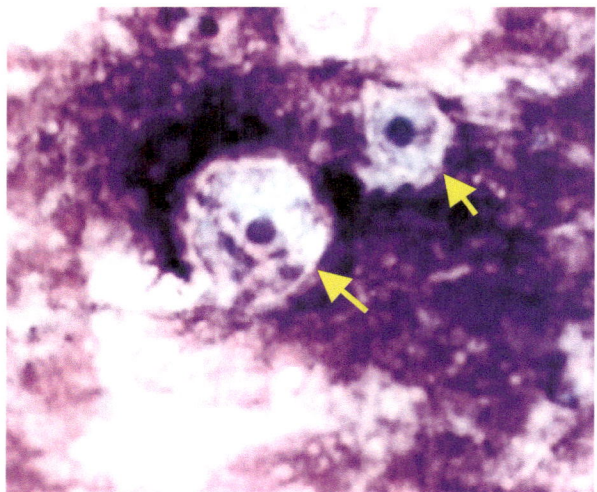

Empty cysts refer to cysts that lose its contents inside the cell, such as the cytoplasm, nucleus, and nucleolus. With Giemsa stain, empty cysts are circular in shape with the double-wall in the color of light blue. The outer layer and inner layer of the double-wall are separated by the transparent gap (Figs. 6.9 and 6.10).

5. Some kinds of cells should be distinguished from *Acanthamoeba* in the smear of the corneal scraping.
   (a) Edematous corneal epithelial cells: The edematous corneal epithelial cells in the corneal smear usually may have the broken cell membrane and a swelling nucleus (Fig. 6.11) or show cytolysis (Fig. 6.12). Although these epithelial

Fig. 6.8 Pre-cyst (shown by black arrow) is spherical in shape with a single-layer wall (Giemsa stain, ×1000)

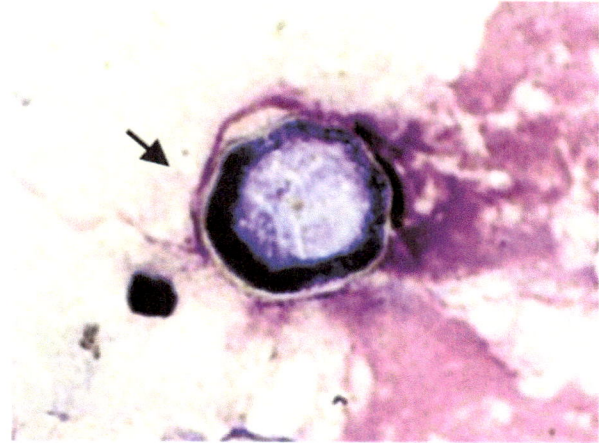

Fig. 6.9 An empty cyst (shown by arrow) is polygonal in shape with double-wall. The cytoplasm, nucleus, and nucleolus are absent (Giemsa stain, ×1000)

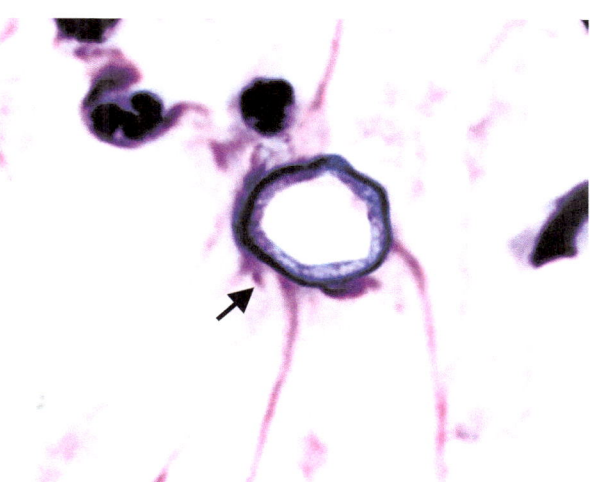

cells have similar size with trophozoites or immature cysts, its nucleus is stained in the color of magenta with the homogenous or plaques nucleoplasm in which one or more nucleoli can be observed.

(b) Inflammatory cells: At early stage and advanced stage of *Acanthamoeba* keratitis, a large amount of neutrophils generally can be observed in the corneal smear. But lymphocytes, mononuclear macrophages are mainly present at later stage of the disease. In addition, eosinophilic granulocytes can be occasionally seen. Because neutrophils and eosinophilic granulocytes contain lobulated nuclei, they are easily distinct from *Acanthamoeba* cyst. Lymphocytes generally are round in shape with little or no cytoplasm and its nuclear is stained in the color of purple-blue without nucleolus. The size of lymphocytes generally is also smaller than that of *Acanthamoeba* cysts. However, some of the activated lymphocytes may contain more cytoplasm

Fig. 6.10 An empty cyst (shown by arrow) still has double-wall in color of light blue (Giemsa stain, ×1000)

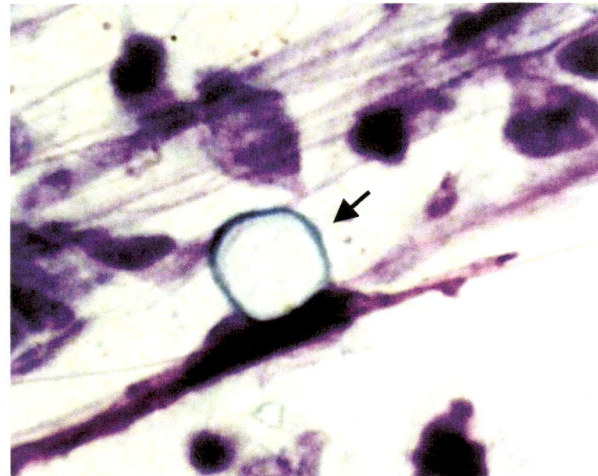

Fig. 6.11 The edematous corneal epithelial cell with the broken membrane and a swelling nucleus (shown by arrow). (Giemsa stain, ×1000)

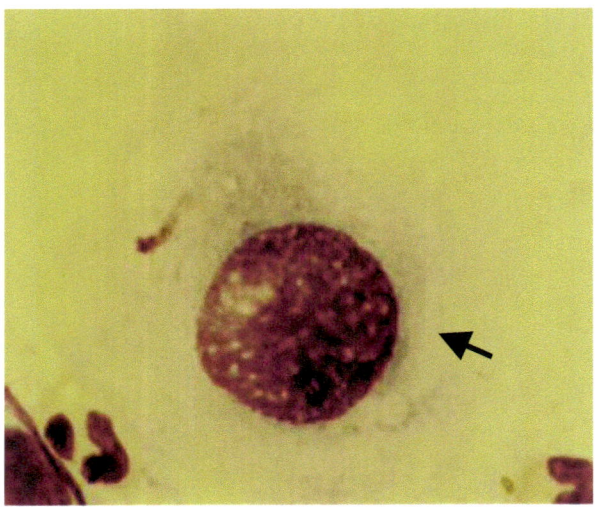

inside the cell and their nucleus is located towards one side of cell with a nucleolus, similar to *Acanthamoeba* cysts. Therefore, activated lymphocytes might be distinguished from *Acanthamoeba* cysts (Fig. 6.13). The mononuclear macrophages have a polymorphic nucleus and contain a large amount of phagocytic particles and vacuoles in the cytoplasm. Hence, they are likely to be confused with *Acanthamoeba* trophozoites (Fig. 6.14).

(c) Swelling hyphae of filamentous fungi: The swelling hyphae of fungi with double-wall structure, which is round in shape, may be observed in the corneal smear. With Giemsa stain, the hyphae of fungi is of blue-purple in color that is surrounded by a transparent shell, but its size is much smaller than that of *Acanthamoeba* cysts (Fig. 6.15).

Fig. 6.12 The corneal epithelial cell (shown by arrow) with cytolysis (Giemsa stain, ×1000)

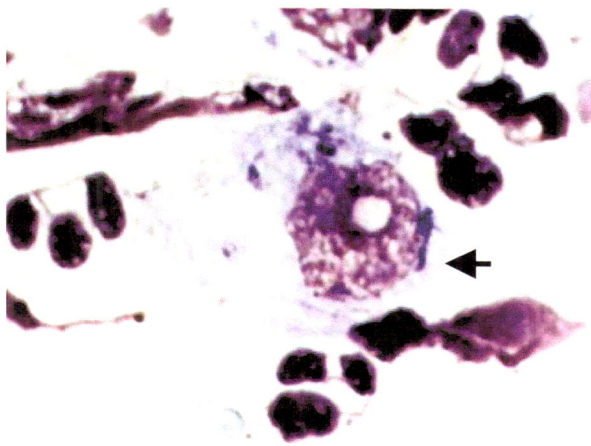

Fig. 6.13 A lymphocyte (shown by red arrow) and an active lymphocyte (shown by black arrow) (Giemsa stain, ×1000)

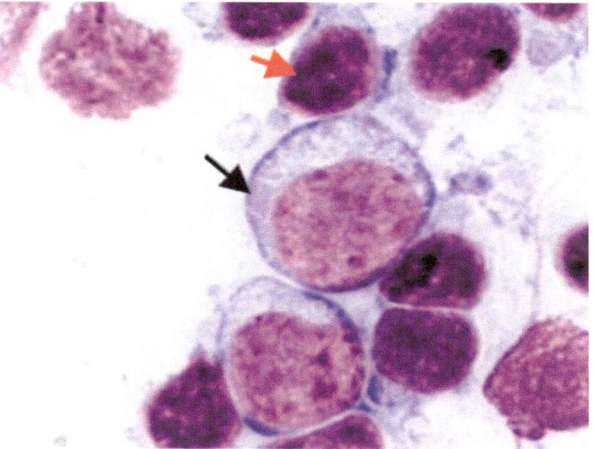

(d) Clusters of necrotic tissues, mucus, and cellulose: Sometimes, mucus and cellulose can form cyst-like structures on the smear examination, but they show various sizes similar to the vacuoles without double-wall and cellular contents. These structures should be differentiated from empty cysts during the smear examination (Fig. 6.16).

(e) Lipid droplets: Generally most of the lipid droplets cannot be stained by Giemsa stain. The lipid droplets on the smear have obvious light refraction with the various sizes, having no cellular contents (Fig. 6.17).

(f) Drug crystallization: The crystals of eye drops are polygonal or amorphous with obvious light refraction on the smear, varying sizes and acellular structure. It is commonly not difficult to differentiate from these crystals of eye drops to *Acanthamoeba* cysts (Fig. 6.18).

Fig. 6.14 A mononuclear macrophage (shown by arrow) with a large amount of phagocytic particles and vacuoles in the cytoplasm (Giemsa stain, ×1000)

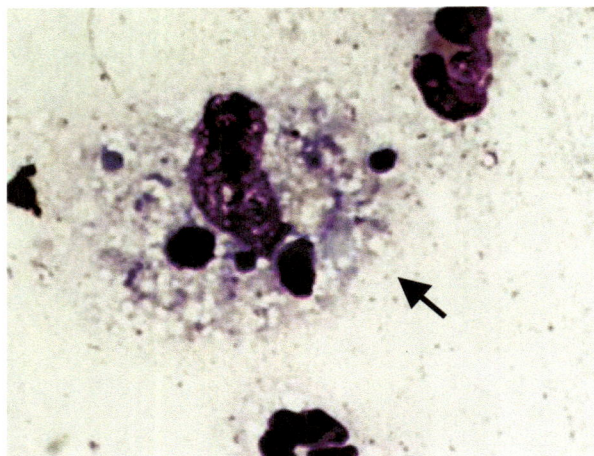

Fig. 6.15 Swelling hyphae of fungi (shown by black arrows) (Giemsa stain, ×1000)

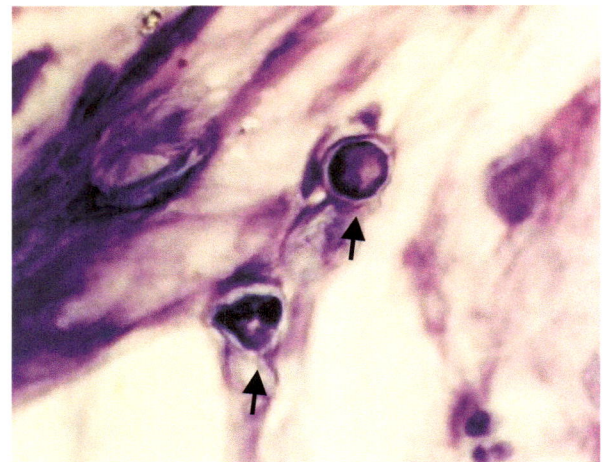

Wet Mount Examination Method

1. Corneal sample collection: The process of the corneal sample collection is as described above.
2. Specimen processing: After instilling 1–2 drops of saline on the surface of a glass slide, the scraped corneal samples are gently smeared on the glass slide. Then the sample on the slide is lightly covered by a glass coverslip and directly submitted to light microscopic examination.
3. Light microscopic examination: In wet mount, *Acanthamoeba* trophozoites are usually in irregular shape due to their mobility, and sometimes migrate between the tissue cells on the smear. In the cytoplasm, there are plenty of coarse particles that vibrate along with the movement of *Acanthamoeba* trophozoites. During the movement of trophozoites, apparent fan-shaped lobopodium, spiny or spear-like protrusions are formed. In the plasma of trophozoites, contractive vacuoles can

Fig. 6.16 A vacuole (shown by red arrow) surrounded by mucus and cellulose (Giemsa stain, ×1000)

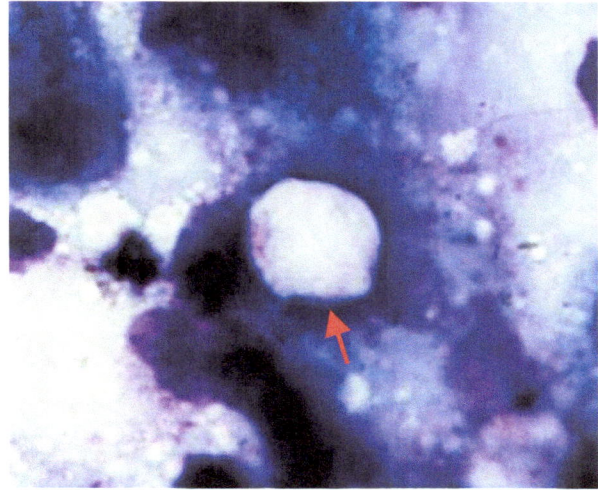

Fig. 6.17 A lipid droplet on the smear (shown by red arrow) without cellular contents (Giemsa stain, ×1000)

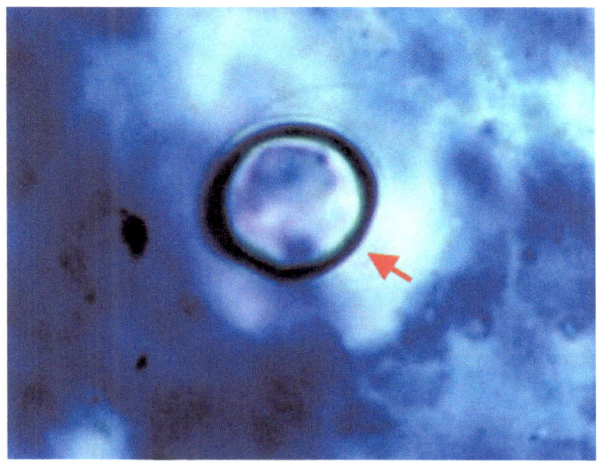

be found that are generally located at one side of the cell. A single nucleus of trophozoite with a large and dense nucleolus surrounded by a transparent zone can be observed (Fig. 6.19).

Mature cysts have a double-wall (Fig. 6.20). The outer layer of the cyst wall is mostly lacy or folded. By contrast, the inner layer is spherical or polygonal. The cyst contains an obvious nucleus with perinuclear halos, and the cytoplasmic granules present immobilization or slight vibratile.

4. *Structures* should be *distinguished* from amoeba.
   (a) Swelling *corneal epithelial cells*: The swelling epithelial cells are often circular in shape and consist of transparent cytoplasm with an oval, large, and dense nucleus with one or more nucleoli. The epithelial cells mostly show clustered and should be distinguished from *Acanthamoeba* cysts, especially from precysts (Fig. 6.21).

Fig. 6.18 The crystallization of eye drops (shown by red arrow) is transparent and polygonal (Giemsa stain, ×1000)

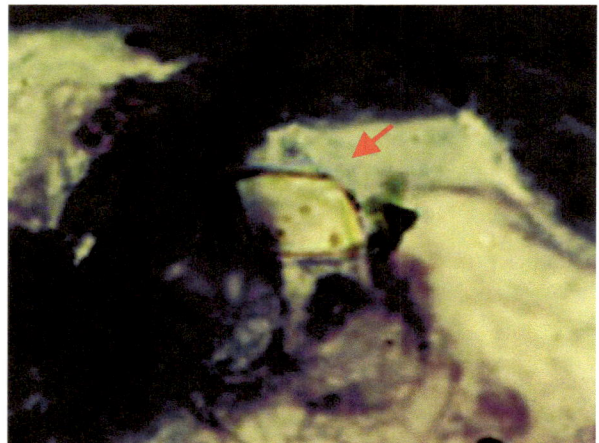

Fig. 6.19 A trophozoite (shown by black arrow) with an obvious nucleus, the porous and coarse particles in the cytoplasm are seen (wet mount, ×1000)

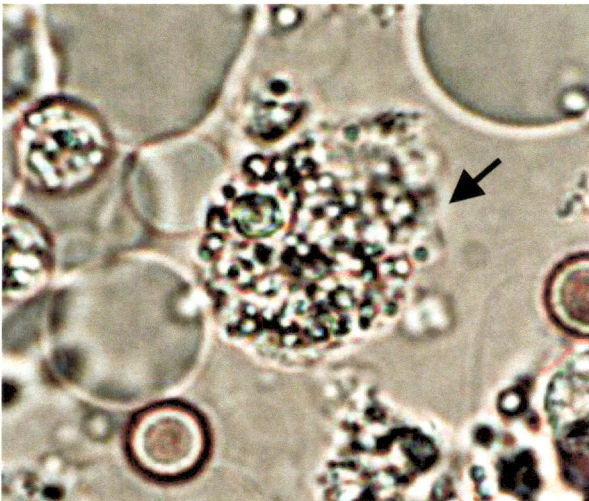

(b) *Monocyte macrophages*: In general, monocyte macrophages are oval in shape and contain rough granular cytoplasm with a large, dense, and oval nucleus (Fig. 6.22).

(c) *Neutrophils*: Neutrophils are circular and slightly smaller in size than that of *Acanthamoeba* cysts and trophozoites. There are lobulated nucleus and sometimes spiculate protuberance that can be seen on the cell membrane. However, neutrophils cannot move between tissue cells on the smear (Fig. 6.23).

(d) Erythrocytes: Erythrocytes, also known as red blood cells, are biconcave, transparent, and reddish with much smaller diameters than that of cysts. Spiculate protuberances can be observed on the membranes of certain shrinking erythrocytes (Fig. 6.24).

Fig. 6.20 A cyst (shown by black arrow) with double-wall. The nucleus and perinuclear halos are obvious (wet mount, ×1000)

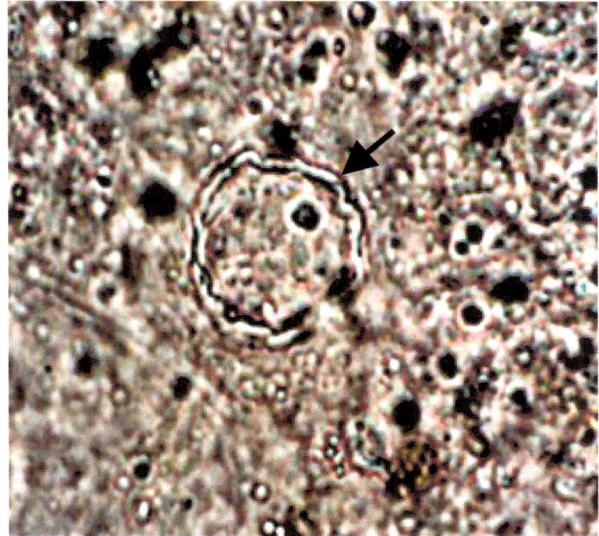

Fig. 6.21 A swelling epithelial cell (shown by black arrow) is oval in shape and contains an oblong nucleus in which a nucleolus is found (wet mount, ×1000)

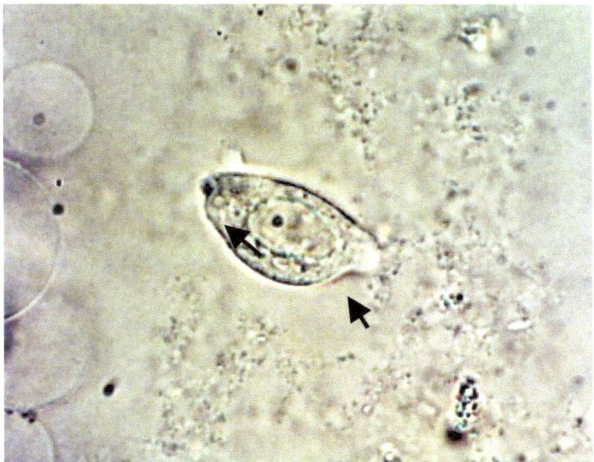

6.2.2   Cultivation of Acanthamoeba

1. Sample collection: Scrapings or the corneal tissue biopsy specimens or other specimens (such as contact lens solution) are collected using sterilized transport swabs (as described above).
2. Culture medium: Page's non-nutrient agar culture medium is used.
3. Inoculation: The Page's non-nutrient agar culture medium plate is prepared and utilized. The suspension of activated or deactivated *E. coli* is applied to the surface of the agar plate. The specimens are inoculated in the center area of the agar plate that is further placed in a wet box and incubated in a 28 °C incubator.

Fig. 6.22 The mononuclear macrophage (shown by black arrow) is oval. An oblong nucleus is present. The cytoplasm contains coarse particles (wet mount, ×1000)

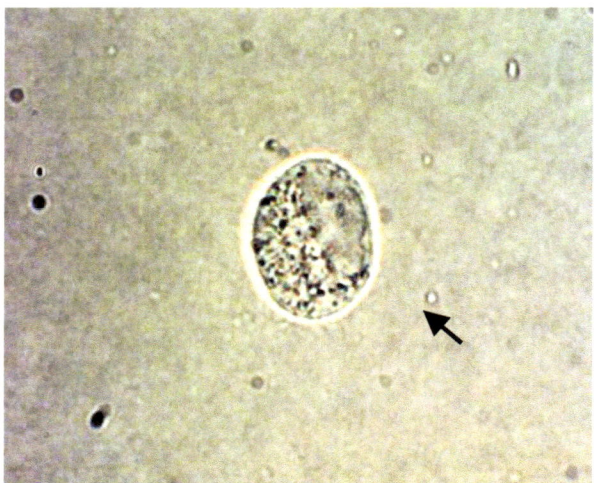

Fig. 6.23 The neutrophil (shown by black arrow) with lobulated nucleus is observed. Spiculate protuberance can be seen on the cell membrane (wet mount, ×1000)

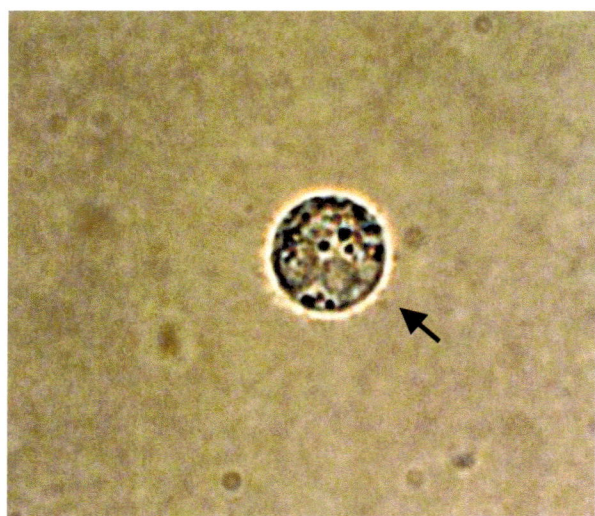

Alternatively, the specimens can also be inoculated in test tubes containing Page's non-nutrient agar culture medium and placed into a 28 °C incubator.

4. Observation with light microscope: The agar culture medium plate is examined every day for up to 10 days for amoeba growth. *Telltale tracks* left by the *migration of amoeba* can be observed in the inoculated position on the surface of the agar plate with low magnification of light microscope (Fig. 6.25). Under light microscope, the trophozoites present circular, oval, or other irregular shapes (Fig. 6.26). The trophozoites can migrate all around for *foraging* on the surface of the agar culture medium plate. Therefore, trophozoites are frequently observed in the *surrounding area* of the inoculation position of the agar plate. The cysts are smaller in size than that of trophozoites and circular or triangular in shape with double-wall. Under light microscope, the cysts show obvious light reflection (Fig. 6.27).

Fig. 6.24 Shrinking erythrocytes (shown by black arrows) are circular with spiculate protuberances on the membrane of cell (wet mount, ×1000)

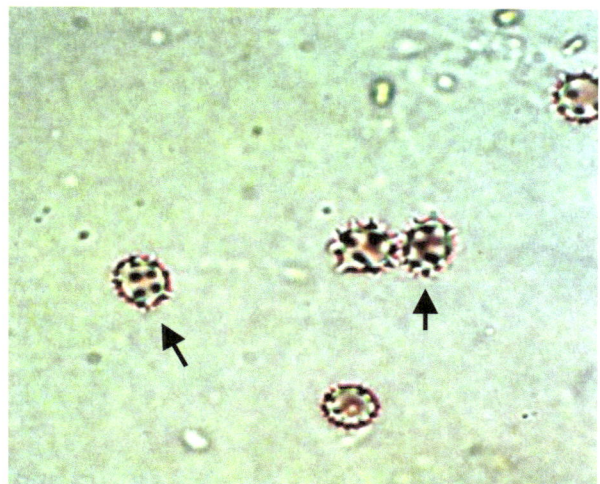

Fig. 6.25 The thin and corrugated traces left by the migration of amoeba on the surface of the agar plate

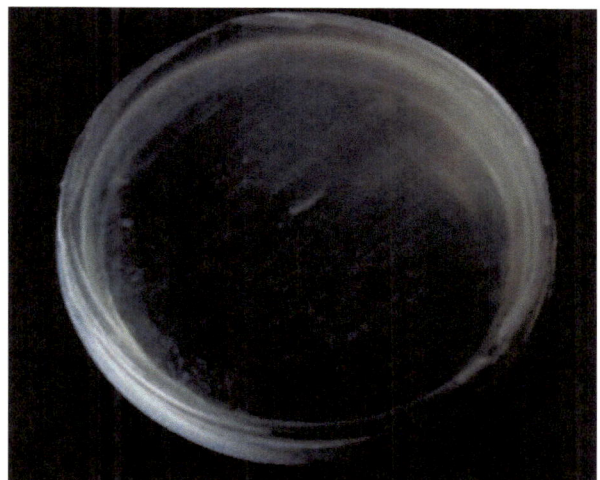

Fig. 6.26 Trophozoites (shown by arrow) that are circular, oval, or have other irregular shapes (×100)

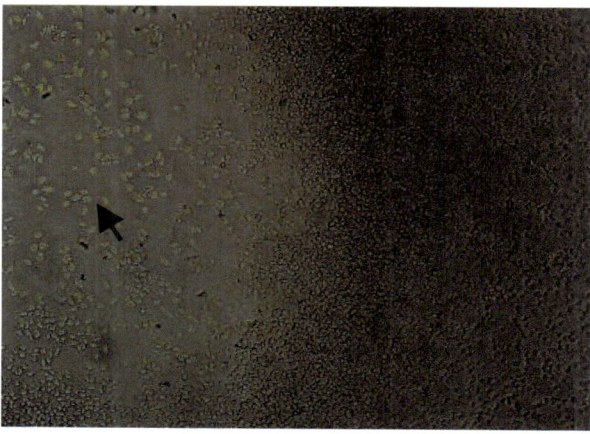

Fig. 6.27 Cysts with obvious light reflection (×100)

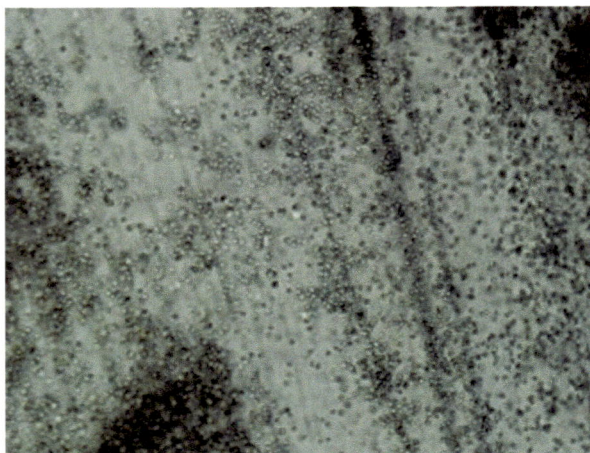

Fig. 6.28 An *Acanthamoeba* trophozoite (shown by arrow) with nucleus, lobopodium, spinous process, and vacuole (×1000)

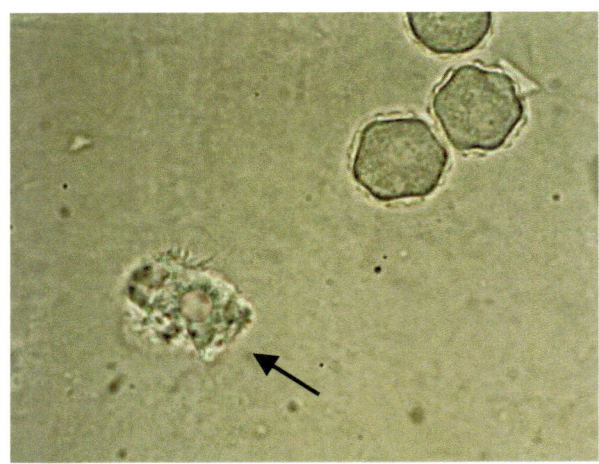

A thin piece of agar on the surface of the *agar plate* is cut using a small blade and observed under a high magnification of light microscope. The form and structure of trophozoites (Fig. 6.28) and cysts (Fig. 6.29) can be clearly seen and distinguished from each other. The nucleus of trophozoites is mostly centered having a diameter of approximately 6 μm. A circular and dense nucleolus is found in the center of the nucleus with a diameter of about 2.4 μm and is surrounded by a transparent strap region. A large amount of lipid droplets, food vacuoles, liquid vacuoles, and other granules are clearly observed in the cytoplasm. Generally, the cysts are circular or quasi-circular with a diameter of 10–25 μm and have relatively thick double-wall. A transparent zone could be seen between the two layers of wall. The outer layer of the wall is often shrinking, whereas the inner layer is smooth and exhibits various shapes, including polygon, circle, star, and triangle. The cytoplasm of cysts is dense and granular and contains obvious nucleus and nucleolus.

Fig. 6.29 Circular cysts (shown by arrow) with thick double-wall. The outer layer of the wall is shrinking, whereas the inner layer of the wall is smooth and polygonal (×1000)

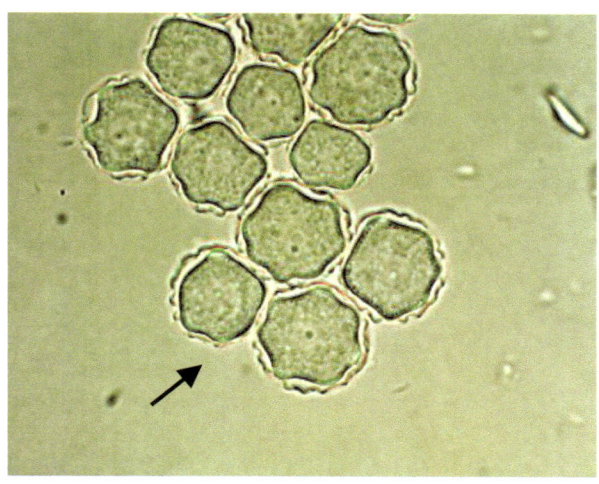

5. Preparation of amoeba culture medium
   (a) The formula of *Page's liquid non-nutrient medium* is

NaCl	120 mg
$MgSO_4 \cdot 7H_2O$	4 mg
$CaCl_2 \cdot 2H_2O$	4 mg
Na_2HPO_4	142 mg
KH_2PO_4	136 mg
Distilled water	1000 mL

The liquid medium is stored in refrigerator at 4 °C after preparation and can be preserved for 3 months.

For the preparation of non-nutrient agar culture medium, 1.5 g agar is added to 100 mL of Page's liquid non-nutrient medium.

(b) The formula of *PYG broth* is

Peptone	10 g
Yeast extract	10 g
Glucose	1 g
NaCl	5 g
L-cysteine	1 g

The above-mentioned agents are dissolved in 1000 mL PBS with pH 7.0 and 0.5 mmol, and are subsequently sterilized by using an autoclave at 121 °C for 15 min or by filtering. Finally PYG broth is stored at 4 °C.

6.2.3   Test of In Vitro Susceptibility to Acanthamoeba

At present, the commonly used in vitro drug sensitivity (or susceptibility) test method in clinical practice is microdilution method.

1. Preparation of culture medium
   (a) Preparation of PYG broth: as described above.
   (b) Preparation of Page's non-nutrient agar medium: as detailed above.
2. Preparation of amoeba strains
   (a) Cultivation of *Acanthamoeba* trophozoites: *Acanthamoeba* trophozoites are obtained from the culture of PYG broth and statically cultured in the incubator at 28 °C for 5–7 days. When the percentage of *Acanthamoeba* trophozoites is more than 95% observed under inverted microscope, the trophozoites can be used for drug sensitivity test.
   (b) Cultivation of *Acanthamoeba* cysts: *Acanthamoeba* trophozoites that are cultured by PYG broth are collected and centrifuged for 5 min (1000 g centrifugal force) in order to adjust the number of trophozoites to 10^6/mL. Then trophozoites are inoculated on a non-nutrient agar plate and statically cultured in the incubator at 28 °C for 7 days. When the percentage of *Acanthamoeba* cysts is more than 95% observed with light microscope, they can be used for drug sensitivity test.
3. *Drug dilution*: Will-be tested drugs are diluted using doubling dilution method according to the commonly used concentration of eye drops in clinical practice.
4. *Drug sensitivity test* method: The PYG broth cultured *Acanthamoeba* trophozoites or cysts in concentration 10^5/mL are inoculated on a 24-well culture plate, respectively, with 2 mL PYG broth in each well. Furthermore, diluted will-be tested drugs are added to wells of the plates for trophozoites or cysts, respectively. In addition, the PYG broth without tested drugs is applied as a blank control. After static culture in the incubator at 28 °C for 24 h, the PYG broth with *Acanthamoeba* are agitated evenly and transferred to centrifuge tubes of 1 mL each which are centrifuged for 5 min with 1000 g centrifugal force. Then the supernatant is discarded and sediments are washed three times using sterile PBS solution. The sediment at the bottom of the centrifuge tubes is transferred and inoculated to non-nutrient agar tubes that contain alive *E. coli*. The agar tubes are statically incubated in the incubator at 28 °C for 14 days. Subsequently, the growth of amoeba is observed under light microscope and the growth rate can be recorded.

   On the basis of the results of the cultivation of *Acanthamoeba* trophozoites or cysts, *the minimum trophozoite amoebicidal concentration (MTAC)* or *minimum cysticidal concentration (MCC)* can be determined. MTAC refers to as the minimum concentration of drug in which amoebic growth is inhibited completely after the co-culture of both the tested drug and trophozoites in the non-nutrient agar tubes. MCC of the tested drug refers to as the minimum concentration of drug in which amoebic growth is inhibited after the co-culture of both the tested drug and cysts in the non-nutrient agar tubes.

6.2.4 Histopathological Examination

When the corneal tissues are deeply invaded by amoeba, the pathogens cannot be easily detected by scraping. The sample can be collected with micro-trephine or from the corneal graft. Pathological section and *H–E stain* is performed after routine tissue fixation. The presence of *Acanthamoeba* cysts or trophozoites can be observed by light microscope (Fig. 6.30). In the corneal tissues cysts of *Acanthamoeba* usually are observed and trophozoites sometimes are seen. Pathogens found by pathological examination are crucial for the confirmation of etiological diagnosis of *Acanthamoeba* keratitis.

6.2.5 Flagellation Test

Flagellation test is mainly used to differentiate *Naegleria fowleri* from *Acanthamoeba. Naegleria fowleri* can transform to a *pear-shaped flagellate* with two or more *flagellae* during a brief transitional stage. *Acanthamoeba* do not transform to flagellate state.

1. Test method: *Acanthamoeba* trophozoites growing on the agar plate are collected by inoculating loop and put in a test glass tube that contains 1 mL of sterile distilled water. The test glass tube is incubated at 37 °C. Two drops of liquid from the test glass tube are extracted after 2 h and 24 h inoculations, respectively, and dropped on the surface of glass slide for the observation with light microscope in high magnification.
2. Identification of results: If 30–50% of the trophozoites transform to a pear-shaped flagellate with two or more of the flagella after 2 h inoculation, and after 24 h inoculation the *flagella* disappeared and trophozoites return to the original form. The flagellation test is identified as positive result, which suggests Naegleria fowleri.

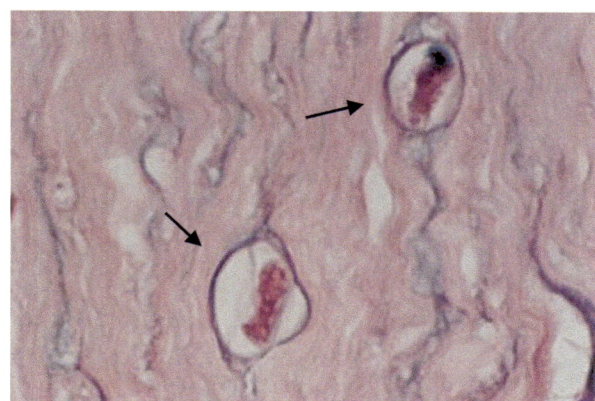

Fig. 6.30 Two *Acanthamoeba* cysts are observed (shown by black arrows) in the biopsy corneal tissue (H–E stain, ×1000)

6.3   Special Examination Methods

6.3.1 *Special Staining* Methods

In order to observe *Acanthamoeba* structures more clearly or in detail, special staining is applied to *Acanthamoeba* which also is useful method for differential diagnosis and clinical research [9].

6.3.1.1 Iodine Tincture Stain

Acanthamoeba trophozoites and cysts can be stained in color of yellow by iodine tincture (Figs. 6.31 and 6.32), which is due to the high content of glycoproteins on the surface of *Acanthamoeba*.

Fig. 6.31 An *Acanthamoeba* cysts stained by iodine tincture (optical microscope ×1000)

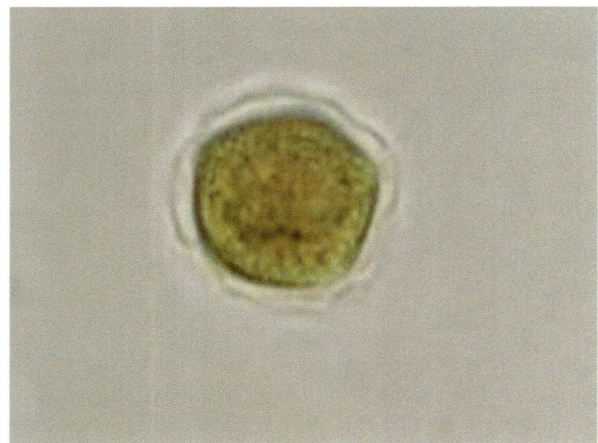

Fig. 6.32 An *Acanthamoeba* trophozoites stained by iodine tincture (optical microscope ×1000)

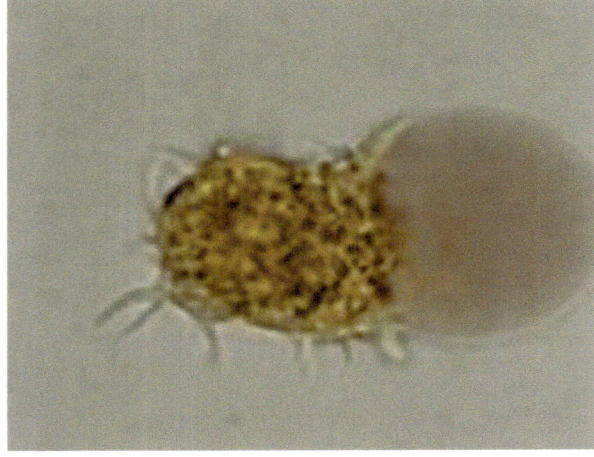

Preparation of iodine tincture solution: iodine (1.0 g) and potassium iodide (2.0 g) are dissolved in 300 mL distilled water.

6.3.1.2 Lactophenol Cotton Blue Stain

Acanthamoeba trophozoites and cysts are stained in the color of blue by lactophenol cotton blue stain. In addition to the stained cyst wall, the thorn-like projections of trophozoites are also stained (Figs. 6.33 and 6.34).

Preparation of lactophenol cotton blue staining solution: crystalline phenol (20 g), lactic acid (20 mL), glycerol (40 mL), and cotton blue (0.05 g) are dissolved in 20 mL distilled water.

6.3.1.3 Fuchsin Stain

Acanthamoeba are colored pale brown by Fuchsin stain. Particularly, the nucleolus is obviously stained, whereas the thorn-like projections are not stained (Figs. 6.35 and 6.36).

Fig. 6.33 An *Acanthamoeba* cyst stained by lactophenol cotton blue stain (optical microscope ×1000)

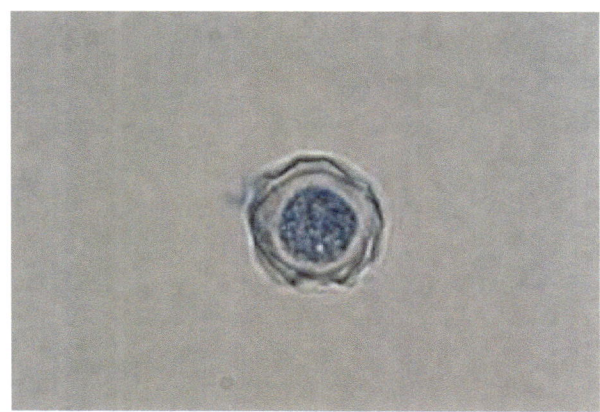

Fig. 6.34 An *Acanthamoeba* trophozoite stained by lactophenol cotton blue stain (×1000)

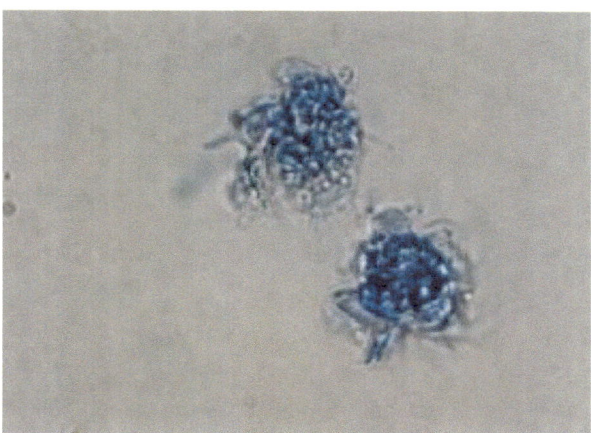

Fig. 6.35 An
Acanthamoeba cyst stained
by Fuchsin stain (×1000)

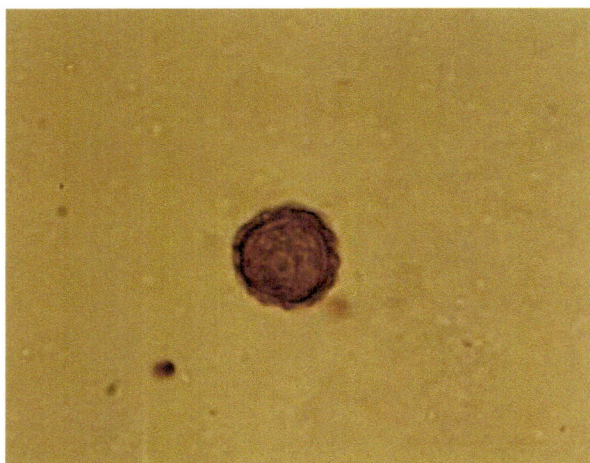

Fig. 6.36 An
Acanthamoeba
trophozoites stained by
Fuchsin stain (×1000)

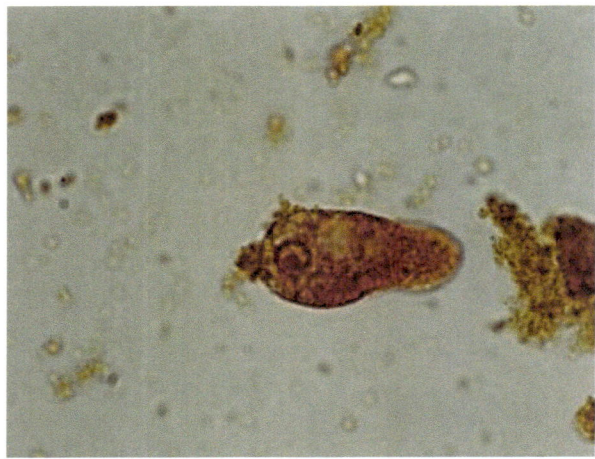

Preparation of Fuchsin staining solution: basic Fuchsin (4 g), alcohol 95% (20 mL), and carbolic acid (8 mL) are dissolved in 100 mL distilled water.

6.3.1.4 Calcofluor White Staining

Calcofluor white stains *Acanthamoeba* in the color of pale blue. The major stained part is the wall of cyst, which is due to the chitin substances of the cyst wall (Fig. 6.37).

Preparation of Calcofluor white staining solution: Calcofluor white (0.1 g) and Evans blue (0.1 g) are dissolved in 100 mL distilled water.

6.3.1.5 Acridine Orange Staining

Acridine orange stains *Acanthamoeba* in color of orange-red (Fig. 6.38).

Acridine orange solution contains acridine orange (1 g) and 802 mL Twain in which 198 mL distilled water is further added. Mcilvaine buffer with pH 3.8 consists of disodium hydrogen phosphate (10.081 g), citric acid monohydrate (13.554 g),

Fig. 6.37 *Acanthamoeba* cysts are stained by Calcofluor white stain (fluorescence microscope ×400)

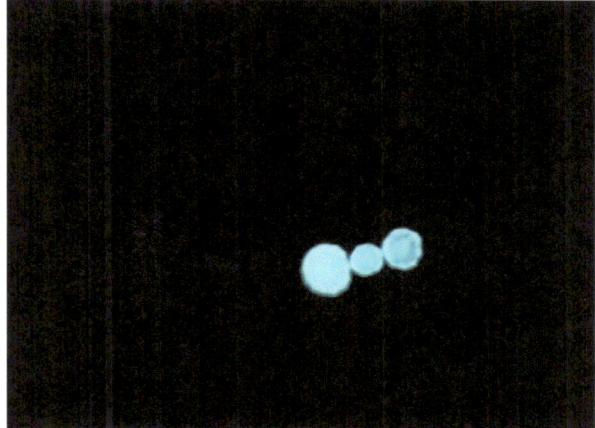

Fig. 6.38 *Acanthamoeba* trophozoites are stained by Acridine orange stain (fluorescence microscope ×400)

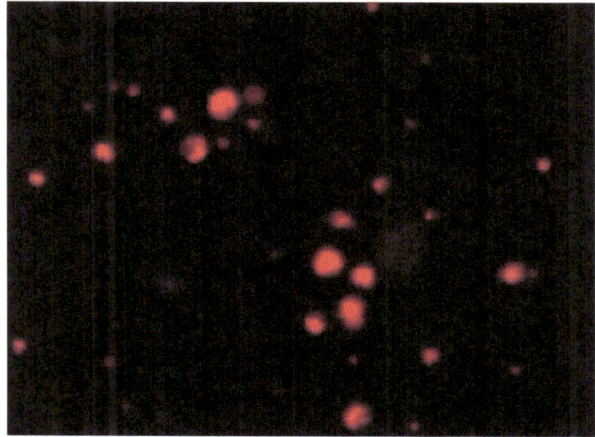

and 1000 mL distilled water. Acridine orange solution and Mcilvaine buffer are preserved and stabilized at −10 °C in 1 year. The working solution is prepared before use by mixing Acridine orange staining solution and Mcilvaine buffer of equal amount (1:1).

Besides, *trypan blue* and *hematoxylin* can also be used for special staining.

6.3.2   Electron Microscope Examination

1. Cultivation of *Acanthamoeba Acanthamoeba* trophozoites or cysts are inoculated in culture dish with built-in *coverslip*. In addition, *Page's non-nutrient liquid medium* and alive *E. coli* are added. The dish is kept in the wet box at 28 °C for incubation for 4 days. After *Acanthamoeba* trophozoites or cysts growing on the surface of the coverslip are observed under optical microscope, the coverslip is taken out and is sent to be processed for observation by scanning electron microscope [10].

2. *Specimen processing* Preparation of specimen for *scanning electron microscope* (SEM): The *Acanthamoeba* growing on the coverslip is fixed using *glutaraldehyde* 2.5% for 12 h and rinsed by 0.1 mol/L PBS solution. Then the specimen is fixed using osmic acid 1% for 1 h and rinsed by tannic acid 2%. Furthermore, the specimen is fixed by osmic acid 1% for a half hour and dehydrated using *gradient ethanol*. Finally, the specimen is saturated by *isoamyl acetate*, and dried at critical point, and sprayed gold in vacuum.

   Preparation of specimen for *transmission electron microscope* (TEM): The corneal tissues are fixed using glutaraldehyde 2.5% for 2 h and rinsed by PBS solution 0.1 mol/L for three times. In addition, the specimen is fixed using osmic acid 1% at 4 °C for 2 h, and dehydrated by a series of ethanol and acetone for six times and saturated by acetone for 2 h. Moreover, the specimen is saturated and embedded by *epoxy resins*. After polymerization, the specimen is sliced into pieces with 40–50 nm and stained by uranyl acetate and lead citrate.

3. Observation of ultrastructure of *Acanthamoeba*

   Characteristics of *Acanthamoeba* under SEM: The diameter of trophozoites is between 15 and 45 μm with quasi-circular, oval, or irregular in shape. On the rough surface of *Acanthamoeba* trophozoites, a large amount of cone-shaped or spinous protuberances can be observed. Lobopodia are extended from the front end of the movement direction of trophozoite.

   The cysts are approximately 10–25 μm in diameter and spherical. The surface of the cysts forms corrugated, honeycomb, or wavy plicae. A number of annular and slightly concave spinous foramens are observed on the surface of the cyst wall. Circular and cap-shaped cover is found within the spinous foramens. Spinous foramen is the exit pathway for the excystation of *Acanthamoeba*. The cover of spinous foramen will dissolve during excystation of *Acanthamoeba*. New *Acanthamoeba* trophozoite (*baby trophozoite*) escapes from the spinous foramen and gradually transforms into mature trophozoite. Subsequently, empty cysts remain after excystation, and circular holes can be found on the cyst wall.

   Characteristics of *Acanthamoeba* under TEM: The cell membrane of the trophozoites can be subdivided into three layers. Free ribosomes, tubule structure, aggregated fibrils, varying amounts of the Golgi apparatus, smooth and rough endoplasmic reticulum, phagocytic vesicles, water vacuoles or contractile vacuoles can be observed in the cytoplasm. In addition, large amounts of mitochondria, lipid droplets, lysosomes, and glycogen granules can be found in the cytoplasm. The wall of cysts exhibits a typical double-layered wall structure. The outer layer of the wall is fibrinous and wrinkled, and displays a parallel network structure. By contrast, the inner layer is smooth and polyhedral that is formed by tenuous fibrils. These two layers are separated by transparent zone. The spinous foramens formed by the fusion of the inner and outer layer of the wall mostly locate at the equatorial zone of the cysts. The spinous foramen of pathogenic *Acanthamoeba* cysts generally present sunken.

6.3.3   Molecular Biology Examination

In recent years, with the rapid development of molecular biotechnology, the molecular biology methods have been expanded and applied in a lot of scientific research fields. Currently, such method has been successfully used for the classification, determination, and *geno-typing* of *Acanthamoeba*. The sensitivity and specificity of the method indicates promising prospect of the application for the etiological diagnosis. However, in clinical applications, the operating steps, experiment conditions, and instruments are needed to be standardized further.

Specific operation method of PCR amplification of *Acanthamoeba 18SrDNA*:

1. *DNA extraction*: The specimen is placed in a 1 mL centrifuge tube. The tube is centrifuged for 15 min at 4000 rpm. The DNA of *Acanthamoeba* is extracted according to the operating steps indicated by the DNA extraction kit (QIAamp DNA Micro Kit). The extracted DNA is stored at −20 °C.
2. *PCR amplification* of 18S rDNA: A gene fragment of around 500 bp is amplified by a pair of *Acanthamoeba* 18SrDNA genotype-specific *primers* JDP1–JDP2. The sequences of the pair of primers are as follows:
   JDP1:5'-GGCCCAGATCGTTTACCGTGAA and JDP2:5'-TCTCACAA GCTGCTAGGGGAGTCA.
3. PCR system (5 μL):

DNA Template	
2*Taq PCR MasterMix Enzyme	25 μL
JDP1	1 μL
JDP2	1 μL
DdH$_2$O	8 μL

4. Parameters of PCR cycle: Firstly, the DNA template is denatured at 95 °C for 7 min. Secondly, the template is subsequently denatured at 95 °C for 60 s, annealed at 62 °C for 45 s and extended at 72 °C for 7 min. Such cycle is repeated for 35 times. Finally, the template is further extended at 72 °C for 5 min.
5. Detection of PCR amplified products: PCR products of 5 μL are extracted in which 6 μL loading buffer is added. Electrophoresis is carried out in agarose gel 1% containing EB (prepared by adding 1.0 g agarose to 100 mL TBE liquid) and operated under 50 V and 14 mA electric current for 40 min. Then the results are observed using the UV lamp (Fig. 6.39).

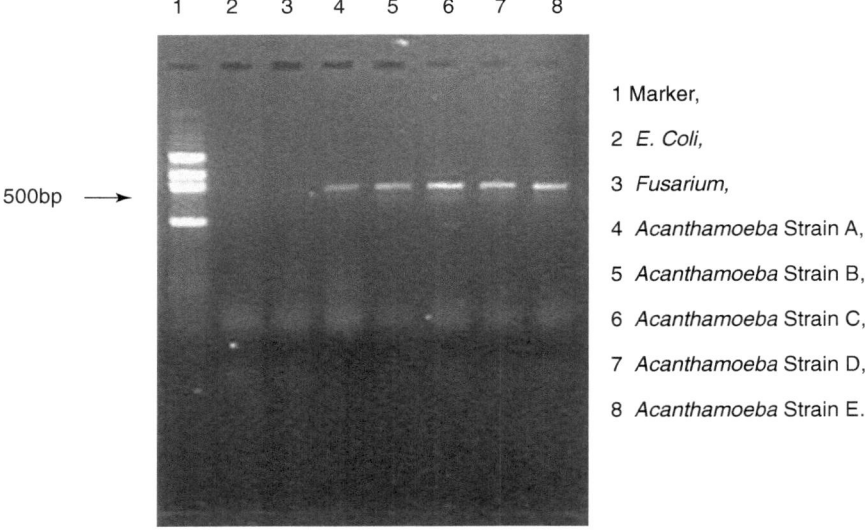

500bp ⟶

1 Marker,

2 *E. Coli,*

3 *Fusarium,*

4 *Acanthamoeba* Strain A,

5 *Acanthamoeba* Strain B,

6 *Acanthamoeba* Strain C,

7 *Acanthamoeba* Strain D,

8 *Acanthamoeba* Strain E.

Fig. 6.39 Electrophoresis result of the product of PCR amplification for *Acanthamoeba*, i.e. a band of approximately 500 bp (serial number of the band is 4–8)

References

1. Wang ZQ, Li R, Zhang C, et al. Morphological characteristics in corneal smear of *Acanthamoeba* keratitis. Zhonghua Yan Ke Za Zhi. 2010;46(5):432–6 [Article in Chinese].
2. Jones DB, Visvesvara GS, Robinson NM. *Acanthamoeba* polyphaga keratitis and *Acanthamoeba* uveitis associated with fatal meningoencephalitis. Trans Ophthalmol Soc U K. 1975;95(2):221–32.
3. Jin X, Luo S, Zhang W, et al. Diagnosis and prevention of *Acanthamoeba* keratitis. Ophthalmology CHN. 1992;1(2):67–71.
4. Luo S, Zhang W, Jin X, et al. The culture and identification of *Acanthamoeba* isolated from the eye. Ophthalmology CHN. 1993;2(4):232–4.
5. Withelmus KR, Osato MS, Font RL, et al. Rapid diagnosis of *Acanthamoeba* keratitis using calcofluor white. Arch Ophthalmol. 1986;104(9):1309–12.
6. Gao W, Cui W, Liu S, et al. Laboratory experiments and clinical diagnosis of *Acanthamoeba* keratitis. Chin J Pract Ophthalmol. 2000;19(11):824–5.
7. Deng X, Pang G, Binji S, et al. Laboratory examination and identification of *Acanthamoeba* isolated from the keratitis. Chin Ophthalmic Res. 1997;15(2):95–7.
8. Deng X, Binji S, Pang G. Laboratory diagnosis and experimental research of *Acanthamoeba* keratitis. Henan Med Res. 2000;9(1):10–3.
9. Gao M, Zhang C, Yang X, et al. Influence of temperatures and pH value on biological activity of *Acanthamoeba* isolated from keratitis. Chin Ophthalmic Res. 2009;27(8):685–7.
10. Luo S, Jin X, Wang Z, et al. Ultrastructure study of pathogen of *Acanthamoeba* keratitis. Chin J Ophthamol. 2008;44(11):1020–4.

7.1 Anti-amoebic Drugs

Currently there are four categories of anti-amoebic drugs that are commonly used in clinical practice for the treatment of *Acanthamoeba* keratitis, including (1) aromatic diamidines, (2) biguanide cationic disinfectants, (3) imidazoles, and (4) aminoglycosides.

7.1.1 Aromatic Diamidines

Aromatic diamidines are one of four categories of anti-amoebic drugs used for treatment of *Acanthamoeba* keratitis, mainly including:

1. Propamidine isethionate
2. Pentamidine isethionate
3. Dibrompropamidine
4. Diminazene aceturate
5. Hydroxystilbamidine isethionate
6. Hexamidine diisethionate

Aromatic diamidines inhibit amoeba by the following possible mechanisms:

1. The effect of *cationic surface activity* generated from the bipolar molecule in diamidines' structure can damage the cell membrane of amoeba cell, which leads to increased cell membrane permeability and the leakage of intracellular ions and biomolecules and further causes the death of amoeba.
2. The diamidines can penetrate into the cells of amoeba, resulting in the *coagulation* and *denaturation* of intracellular structural proteins and directly interfering in the synthesis of nucleic acids.

© Springer Nature Singapore Pte Ltd.
& People's Medical Publishing House, PR of China 2018
X. Sun, *Acanthamoeba Keratitis*, https://doi.org/10.1007/978-981-10-5212-5_7

3. The amount of drugs which connected to the membrane of amoeba cell is cor-
related with the length of alkyl chain in the molecular structure of the diamidines. The longer alkyl chain increases lipophilicity, makes the connection
between the diamidines and lipid bilayer structure easier, and rapidly enhances
the concentration of drugs in the cell that enables to kill amoeba. For example,
the effect of *killing amoeba* of hexamidine (with six alkyl groups) is stronger
than that of propamidine (with three alkyl groups) in vitro and in vivo [1, 2].

Diamidines can also promote the *transformation* of *Acanthamoeba* trophozoites
to cysts, which easily results in increasing drug resistance of amoeba. Such phe-
nomenon might be related to the fact that diamidines could affect the metabolism
level of amebic *intracellular polyamines* or interfere with the *synthesis of polyamines* [3, 4]. Moreover caution should be taken about the toxicity on the corneal
epithelium resulting from the long-term use of diamidines during the treatment [5].

Currently there are two types of *commercial medicine products* of aromatic
diamidines applied in clinical practice, i.e., 0.1% propamidine isethionate eye drops
and ointments (brand name *Brolene*) and 0.1% hexamidine diisethionate (brand
name *Desomedine*).

7.1.2 Cationic Biguanide Disinfectants

Cationic biguanide disinfectants in clinical practice for the treatment of
Acanthamoeba keratitis mainly include:

1. Chlorhexidine
2. Polyhexamethylene biguanide (PHMB)

According to the results of in vitro drug sensitivity test and clinical therapeutic
efficacy, chlorhexidine and PHMB are considered as the most effective drugs for
killing *Acanthamoeba* trophozoites and cysts (*trophozoitocide* and *cystocide*) and
are first choice of anti-*Acanthamoeba* drugs in clinical treatment. The anti-amoebic
effects of cationic biguanide disinfectants mainly depend on the affecting the function of amoeba cell membrane [6]. After interacting with chlorhexidine or PHMB,
the contents of *Acanthamoeba* cysts shrink, and the wall of the cyst becomes edematous and swollen. In addition, PHMB causes more apparent changes in the structure of cysts, including the reduction of the cytoplasm, the occurrence of large
amounts of high-density clustered sediments on the cell surface, the aggregation of
nuclear chromatin, and the overflow of *intranuclear contents*.

Compared with PHMB, chlorhexidine mainly interferes with the cytoplasm of
cysts and hardly involves in the components of the nucleus [7, 8]. The minimum
cysticidal concentration (MCC) of chlorhexidine is 0.49–15.6 µg/ml, while, for
PHMB, the MCC is 0.49–3.9 µg/ml. When chlorhexidine eye drop 0.02% is applied
on the ocular surface, the concentration of the drug can reach to 1.218 µg/g in rabbit
corneal tissues [9].

Commonly these are the *therapeutic concentrations* of cationic biguanide disinfectants used in clinical practice: chlorhexidine 0.02% (200 µg/ml) and 0.04% (400 µg/ml) and PHMB 0.02% (200 µg/ml) and 0.04% (400 µg/ml). It was reported in a literature that the concentration of both drugs can be increased to 0.06% for severe cases [10].

It has been confirmed by in vitro experiments that chlorhexidine 0.02% and PHMB 0.02% show relatively low *toxicity* to the corneal epithelial cells. Particularly, the ability of nonspecific binding of chlorhexidine with the corneal tissue is rather low [11]. But when the concentration of drug is more than 0.2%, cationic biguanide disinfectants can cause apparent toxicity on the conjunctival and the corneal epithelial cells.

Up to now there are no commercial cationic biguanide eye drop products available in the market. The eye drops of cationic biguanide mentioned above are usually hospital-made (the *pharmaceutical formulation* is introduced in detail in Sect. 7.5).

7.1.3 Imidazoles

Imidazoles are broad-spectrum antifungal agents and generally used in combination with cationic biguanide disinfectants. Imidazoles used in clinical practice mainly include:

1. Ketoconazole
2. Fluconazole
3. Miconazole
4. Clotrimazole

Imidazoles competitively inhibit the lanosterol 14α-demethylase in cell membrane, leading to the accumulation of *lanosterols* and inhibition of the *biosynthesis* of *ergosterol* in cell membrane. Subsequently, the permeability of cell membrane is influenced, resulting in the death of the pathogens. However, with the concentration commonly used in clinical practice, imidazoles can only inhibit the activity of amoeba and cannot directly kill the pathogens. The minimum trophozoite amoebicidal concentration (MTAC) of ketoconazole is 144 µg/ml, and the minimum cysticidal concentration (MCC) of ketoconazole is above 500 µg/ml. After oral ketoconazole, the drug concentration within the corneal tissues only reaches to 0.5 µg/g, which is far below the MTAC and MCC. Therefore, ketoconazole is not frequently applied alone in clinical practice. The minimum trophozoite amoebicidal concentration (MTAC) of fluconazole is 320 µg/ml [8].

The concentration of imidazoles *eye drops* commonly used for clinical treatment is 1%. It has been confirmed in a study that the drug concentration within the corneal tissue is 200–250 µg/g after applying itraconazole eye drop 1% [12]. When oral administration of itraconazole was used, the drug concentration within the corneal tissues is only 0.05 µg/g [13]. Furthermore, oral administration of itraconazole may result in several side effects. Generally imidazoles eye drop may only be used in combination therapy with cationic biguanide disinfectants during the treatment of *Acanthamoeba* keratitis.

7.1.4   Aminoglycosides

Aminoglycoside commonly used in clinical practice for the treatment of *Acanthamoeba* keratitis mainly include:

1. Neomycin
2. Paromomycin

Aminoglycosides predominantly inhibit the synthesis of *bacterial protein* and affect the *permeability* of bacterial outer membrane. As for the effectiveness of anti-amoeba, aminoglycosides mainly interfere with the function of the cell membrane of amoeba. Paromomycin was a drug initially used in the treatment of *Entamoeba histolytica*, which showed good clinical effect. However, its effect on *Acanthamoeba* keratitis is not satisfactory [14]. In vitro experiments have showed that aminoglycosides have strong lethal effect on trophozoites but poor effect on cysts. The in vitro MCCs of neomycin and paromomycin are above 500 µg/ml [15]. The concentration of neomycin eye drops in clinical application is 0.5%. In clinical practice, aminoglycoside drugs are generally used in combination with cationic biguanide disinfectants [16].

7.1.5   Drug Susceptibility

Amoebas at different growing phases show varying degrees of drug sensitivity. Studies reported that the descending order of the susceptibility of amoebas to chlorhexidine is as follows: amoebic precysts, trophozoites at logarithmic growth phase, and mature cysts. But the susceptibility of trophozoites at logarithmic growth phase to PHMB is higher than that of amoebic precysts and mature cysts [17].

According to the difference in drug susceptibility of amoebas at different phases, the regimen of therapy commonly used in clinical practice is the combination therapy, i.e., two or more types of anti-amoebic drugs mentioned above are combined for the treatment. In vitro investigations of anti-amoebic drugs showed that cationic biguanide disinfectants have synergistic effect with diamidines or neomycin. Cationic disinfectants damage the cell membrane of amoeba and help diamidines or neomycin penetrate the membrane of the cell, which enables diamidines or neomycin to interact with intracellular enzymes, structural proteins, and nucleic acids more effectively and further shows the lethal effect [18]. Different combinations of anti-amoebic drugs, including PHMB with propamidine, PHMB with chlorhexidine, propamidine with neomycin, polymyxin B, gramicidin, etc., obtain satisfactory clinical efficacy [19–21]. In clinical studies of about 150 patients with *Acanthamoeba* keratitis, with different combinations of anti-amoebic drugs, i.e., *chlorhexidine 0.02% and neomycin 0.5% or chlorhexidine 0.02%, neomycin 0.5%*, and *metronidazole 2%* eye drops, the clinical therapeutic effects were satisfactory [22–24].

7.1.6   Effect of Glucocorticoids

Glucocorticoids originally have no inhibition effect on amoeba pathogens. As for the application of glucocorticoids in the therapy of *Acanthamoeba* keratitis, there are different opinions. In vitro experiments indicated that glucocorticoids can promote the proliferation of *Acanthamoeba* trophozoites, increase the virulence of amoebas [25], inhibit the *phagocytic activity* of macrophages of the host, and further affect the clearance of amoebas from the corneal tissues [26]. The results of animal experiments showed that the use of glucocorticoids could aggravate the severity of *Acanthamoeba* keratitis [27] and increase the duration of treatment [28].

However, some of the studies showed that glucocorticoids can impede the transformation of trophozoites into cysts, which may enhance the *amoebicide effect* of drugs. After treatment with amoebicide drugs for 1 or 2 weeks, with improved condition of keratitis, moderate doses of glucocorticoids can effectively reduce the damage of the corneal tissues. Therefore, the combination therapy using both amoebicide drugs and glucocorticoids is considered to be safe for clinical practice [29]. Clinical reports also showed that the combination of amoebicides and *immunosuppressants* such as glucocorticoids, cyclophosphamide, and azathioprine for the treatment of severe amoebic scleritis could effectively relieve pains of the patients and reduce the tissue damage [30].

On the basis of our clinical data and the experiences in treatment of *Acanthamoeba* keratitis, we suggest that topical glucocorticoids can aggravate infection and induce the recurrence of *Acanthamoeba* keratitis (Figs. 7.1 and 7.2) and in some cases topical glucocorticoids result in indolent corneal ulceration. Therefore, topical glucocorticoids should be avoided until the pathogens are not detected by repeat smear of the corneal scraping or by repeat corneal confocal microscopy examinations.

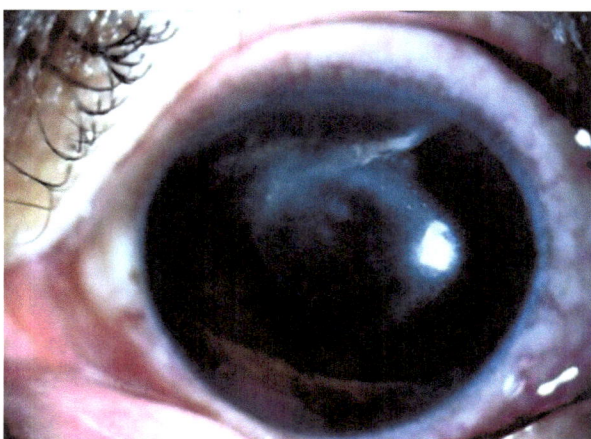

Fig. 7.1 *Acanthamoeba* keratitis for 1 month. The infiltration corneal stroma, without the corneal ulcer

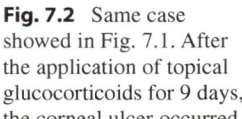

Fig. 7.2 Same case showed in Fig. 7.1. After the application of topical glucocorticoids for 9 days, the corneal ulcer occurred

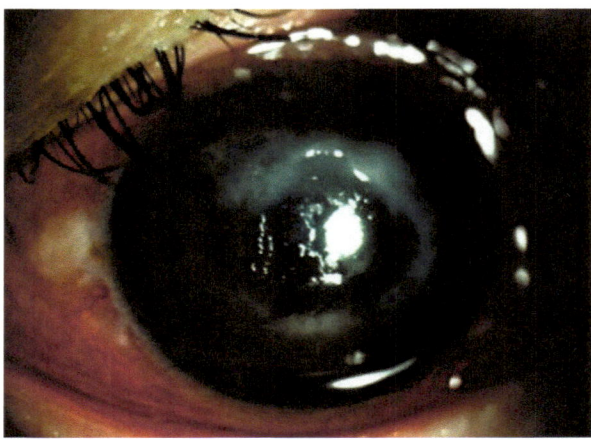

7.1.7 Novel Anti-amoebic Drugs Investigated

1. Alkylphosphocholines (APCs)
APCs were initially investigated as antitumor drugs [31]. At present, APCs are found to have good lethal effect on protozoa, such as *Leishmania*, *Trypanosoma cruzi*, and *Entamoeba histolytica*. It has been confirmed that APCs may achieve the lethal effect mainly by damaging the cell membrane of amoeba [32]. One of the major representative drugs is miltefosine. It was observed in vitro that the treatment of 80 μM miltefosine for 1 hour can kill nearly 100% of the trophozoites and 160 μM miltefosine can kill 90% of the cysts. With low concentration such as 5 μM, miltefosine could effectively inhibit the transformation of cysts into trophozoites.

2. Methylglyoxal-Bis(guanylhydrazone) (MGBG)
MGBG also is an antitumor drug. It primarily is applied to impede the proliferation of amoeba through the inhibition of ornithine decarboxylase. Because MGBG shows weak and reversible inhibition against S-adenosylmethionine decarboxylase, MGBG can induce the transformation of trophozoites into cysts. The drug concentration of MGBG that effectively inhibit amoebas in vitro is 1 mM [33].

3. Povidone Iodine
Povidone iodine is a chemical complex of polyvinylpyrrolidone and iodine and has rapid and broad-spectrum effects against bacteria, fungus, and virus. Due to the hydrophilicity of povidone, iodine can be delivered to the carrier of the cell membrane. As a consequence, the free iodine released can rapidly induce cytotoxicity and kill the cell. Studies showed that povidone iodine from 0.5% to 2.5% has good lethal effects on trophozoites and cysts, while povidone iodine 1.0% has no toxicity on the corneal epithelium and endothelium [34, 35].

4. Myristamidopropyl Dimethylamine (MAPD)

MAPD is a cationic disinfectant and shows good lethal effect on bacteria, fungi, and amoebas. The in vitro anti-amoebic mechanism of this drug still remains unclear. The MCC of MAPD ranges from 6.25 to 25 μg/ml. One of the characteristics of MAPD is its small molecular weight (300 Da). By contrast, molecular weights of chlorhexidine and PHMB are 898 Da and 2340 Da, respectively. Therefore, it is likely that MAPD has better penetration and higher drug concentration in the corneal tissues [36–38].

5. Caspofungin

Caspofungin is a member of a new class of echinocandin B antifungal drug. It has noncompetitive inhibition of against β-(1,3)-glucan synthase, interferes with the synthesis of β-(1,3)-glucan in the fungal cell wall, and leads to change the cell wall structure, further causing cell rupture. The anti-amoebic mechanism of caspofungin is currently unclear. It has been shown that 250 mg/L caspofungin can effectively kill trophozoites, and 500 mg/L caspofungin has a lethal effect on cysts [39, 40].

6. Artemisinin

Artemisinin is a new type of antimalarial drug extracted from *Artemisia annua* and is also the preferred drug for the treatment of cerebral malaria and falciparum malaria. Its derivatives include dihydroartemisinin, artemether, arteether, and artesunate, and all of its derivatives contain a peroxide bridge structure, which can generate large amounts of free radicals and reactive oxygen in vivo by cleavage, and inhibit the growth of plasmodium and damage the structure of cell membrane. In vitro studies confirmed that artesunate could inhibit the proliferation of amoebas. In addition, the inhibition effect on amoeba by artesunate is concentration-dependent [41, 42].

The effects of all novel anti-amoebic drugs mentioned above are predominantly based on the in vitro experiments. Their clinical efficacy on *Acanthamoeba* keratitis still needs to be further investigated.

7.2   Clinical Therapeutic Principles and Regimens

7.2.1   Therapeutic Principles

1. In clinical practice, the therapeutic regimens should be selected according to different stages (early, advanced, and late stages) and severity of the disease.
2. The combined drug therapy is considered firstly. Generally two or three types of anti-amoebic drugs are selected for combined therapeutic regimen.
3. The duration of drug therapy requires more than 6 months.
4. Surgical management should be timely applied when drug therapy is invalid. After surgery, anti-amoebic medicines are continued for at least 3 months.

7.2.2   Therapeutic Regimens

1. Treatment for Patients at Early Stage

Because the corneal lesion at early stage is usually limited to the epithelial layer or the corneal shallow stroma, the therapy with topical anti-amoebic drugs is the first choice generally. Chlorhexidine 0.02% or PHMB 0.02% with neomycin 0.5% or metronidazole 2% can be selected for combined drug treatment. During the initial treatment, eye drops of anti-amoebic drugs should be applied hourly day and night for at least 1–2 weeks. Then eye drops are administered once per hour during the day with tobramycin eye ointment or fusidic acid eye gel at night. According to the efficacy of treatment, eye drops are tapered gradually from once every 2 hours to two times a day.

For patients with the corneal shallow stromal ulcer, the debridement of the corneal lesions can be carried out for one or two times in a week, which is helpful for the penetration of anti-amoebic medicines and the reduction of amounts of pathogens. (Figs. 7.3 and 7.4). After debridement of the corneal lesion, antibiotic eye drops have to be used for prophylaxis of bacterial infection. For example, levofloxacin or gatifloxacin eye drops usually are selected for three to four times per day, and antibiotic ointment will be used at night.

Cautery with iodine tincture 5% once a week is recommended for patients with corneal shallow stromal ulcer. It is suggested that cautery with iodine tincture 5% should not be frequently applied in order to avoid the aggravation of the anterior chamber reaction and the serious pain of patients.

During the therapy, topical antiglaucoma drugs should be given in time if increased intraocular pressure is found. For patients with severe eye pain, oral administration of analgesics or sedative drugs can be considered, which is beneficial for patients to rest at night and compliance of topical anti-amoebic drug treatment.

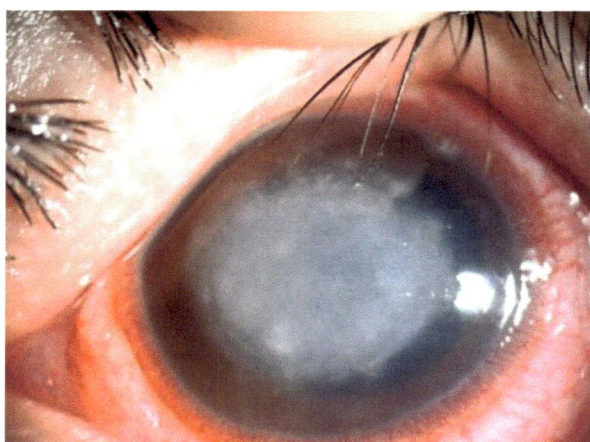

Fig. 7.3 *Acanthamoeba* keratitis in the right eye for 2 months before the anti-amoebic treatment

Fig. 7.4 One month after anti-amoebic drug treatment, with debridement of the corneal lesion and cautery with iodine tincture 5%, the corneal nebula was formed (the same patient in Fig. 7.3)

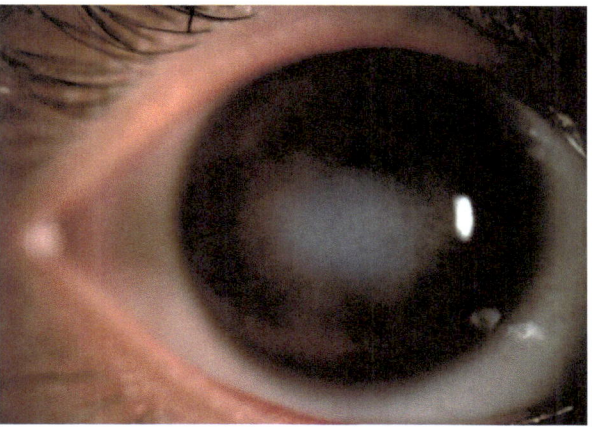

2. Treatment for Patients at Advanced Stage and Later Stage

For patients at advanced stage, besides the topical anti-amoebic drugs, oral terbinafine (250 mg/day) or itraconazole (100–200 mg/day) could be administered for 1–2 weeks. If the corneal ulcer is progressive or with obvious hypopyon in anterior chamber, surgical management should be needed as soon as possible.

For patients at late stage, the corneal surgery has to be carried out immediately. After the surgery, eye drops of cyclosporine A 1% or tacrolimus 0.1% can be used (two to four times a day usually) with topical anti-amoebic drug therapy for at least 3 months. Topical glucocorticoid should not be used in 1 month after surgery.

7.3   Surgical Management

7.3.1   Debridement and Cautery of the Corneal Ulcer

1. Debridement method for corneal ulcer: after topical anesthesia is applied, the eyelids are opened by an eye speculum to expose the corneal lesion. The discharges on the surface of the corneal ulcer are wiped clean with dry cotton swabs. In addition, the necrotic tissues on the surface should be scraped, with a surgical small round blade or curette. Subsequently, the surface of the corneal ulcer is cauterized by iodine tincture 5%.
2. Cauterization method by iodine tincture 5%: after the debridement of the corneal ulcer, iodine tincture 5% is applied with a cotton swab for cauterization on the surface of the corneal ulcer area. The time of cauterization should be limited to approximately 20 s. Then the surface of the corneal ulcer area is flushed with sterile saline solution for about 30–60 s (Figs. 7.5 and 7.6).

During the process of debridement, the edge of the curette should be parallel to the surface of the corneal ulcer, and deep curettage should be avoided. If patients

Fig. 7.5 *Acanthamoeba* keratitis for 2 months. The corneal ulcer, ring infiltration, and hypopyon in anterior chamber were observed before the treatment

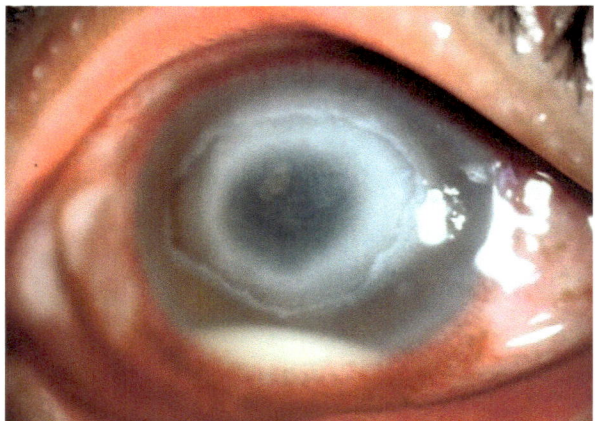

Fig. 7.6 After treatment with the topical anti-amoebic medicine, debridement, and cautery, the corneal ulcer was healed (the same patient in Fig. 7.5) and hypopyon disappeared

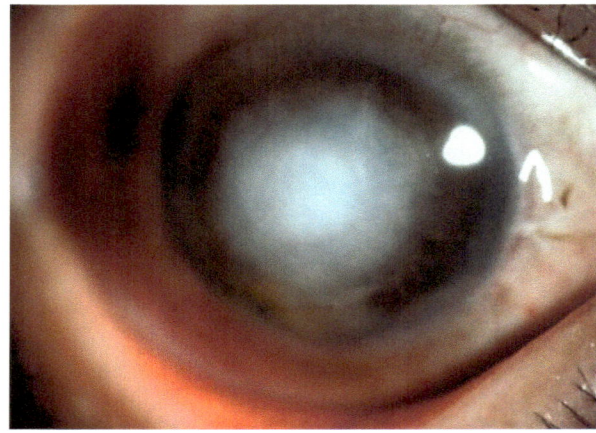

have the tendency of descemetocele or perforation of the cornea, debridement of the corneal ulcer is contraindicated. The debridement treatment could also be combined with amniotic membrane transplantation.

The appropriate frequency of cauterization with iodine tincture 5% is one or two times per week in order to avoid protracting the healing of the ulcer and aggravating inflammatory reaction of anterior chamber.

7.3.2   Excision of Necrotic Tissues of the Corneal Lesions and Amniotic Membrane Transplantation

After 2-3 weeks of the therapy with eye drops of anti-amoebic medicines, if the corneal ulcer still progresses, or if there are still many *Acanthamoeba* cysts in the corneal tissues observed through the corneal confocal microscope or by the smear examination of the corneal scraping, the excision of the corneal lesions combined with the amniotic membrane transplantation can be indicated in order to reduce the amount of pathogens and diminish the inflammation in the corneal tissues.

1. *Excision of the corneal lesions*: after topical anesthesia is applied, the eyelids are opened by an eye speculum. The necrotic tissues of the corneal lesions are excised with a sharp knife. Then cauterization with iodine tincture 5% is used. If the depth of excision of the corneal lesion exceeds 1/4 of the corneal stroma, amniotic membrane transplantation should be combined in order to avoid protracting the healing of the corneal ulcer after the excision.

2. *Amniotic membrane transplantation*: after topical anesthesia is applied, the eyelid is opened by an eye speculum. The necrotic tissues on the surface of the corneal ulcer are scraped. Edema epithelial cells around the corneal lesion area are eliminated. After the excision of the corneal lesions and cauterization with iodine tincture 5%, two to four layers of amniotic membrane are clipped. The surface of the corneal ulcer is covered by amniotic membrane of which the diameter is 3 mm larger than that of the corneal ulcer area. Furthermore, 10-0 nylon monofilament is applied for interrupted suture. Bandage corneal contact lens is used after the surgery (Figs. 7.7a–d and 7.8a–d).

After the surgery, the patients should be followed every day in 1 week. Topical anti-amoebic drug treatment is continued. In addition, the antibiotic and nonsteroidal anti-inflammatory eye drops can be added in order to reduce the inflammation and prevent the bacterial infection.

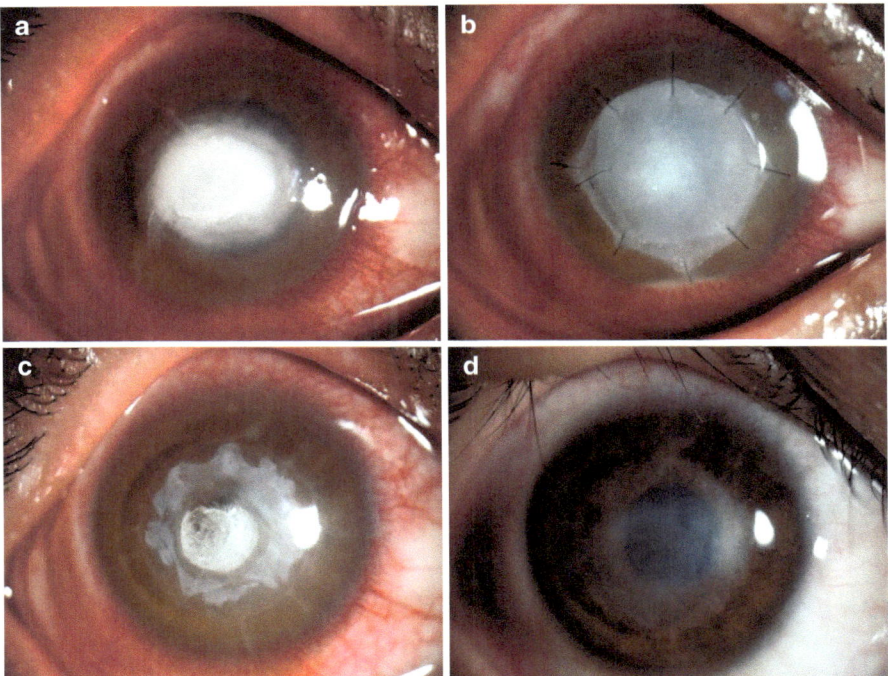

Fig. 7.7 (**a**) The corneal ulcer of a patient with *Acanthamoeba* keratitis for 1 month before surgery treatment. (**b**) After the excision of the corneal lesion, combined with fresh amniotic membrane transplantation. (**c**) One month after the surgery, most of the amniotic membrane was resolved, and the ulcer was healed mostly. A half year after surgery, the corneal nebula was formed

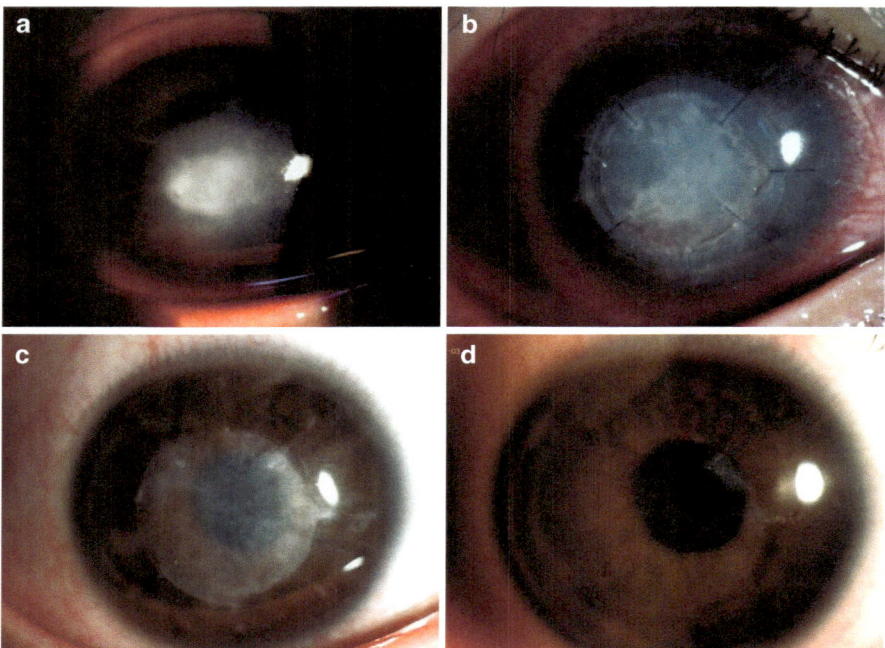

Fig. 7.8 (**a**) The corneal ulcer of a patient with *Acanthamoeba* keratitis for 2 months before the surgery. (**b**) One day after the excision of the corneal lesion, combined with frozen-dry amniotic membrane transplantation. (**c**) Three months after the surgery, the corneal ulcer was healed and amniotic membrane transplanted was partially resolved. (**d**) Three years after the surgery, the mild corneal nebula was formed, and the uncorrected visual acuity was 15/20

Because the frozen-dry amniotic membrane remains transparent after rehydration and transplantation, which is beneficial to observing the changes of the corneal lesions after the surgery, it is preferred to use the frozen-dry amniotic membrane for the transplantation. Before surgery, chlorhexidine eye drops 0.02% could be used to rinse the amniotic membrane for 10–15 min. Thus, the amniotic membrane can play the role of drug delivery system after transplantation. The bandage contact lens should be used after the surgery, which can reduce the absorbing of the amniotic membrane. The therapy with topical anti-amoebic drugs should be continued for at least 3 months after the surgery.

7.3.3 Corneal Transplantation

The corneal transplantation should be considered for patients at advanced or late stage.

1. *Lamellar corneal transplantation*: If anti-amoebic medicine therapy is not effective and the corneal lesions invaded into the deep corneal stroma, lamellar corneal transplantation is indicated. The depth of the corneal lesions should be carefully observed by the slit lamp before operation in order to determine the depth of the corneal stroma to be excised.

Fig. 7.9 The corneal ulcer
of *Acanthamoeba* keratitis
for 2 months

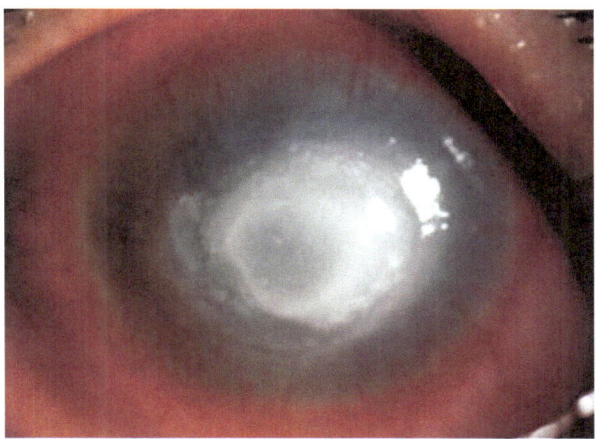

Fig. 7.10 A year after
penetrating keratoplasty
with clear graft cornea

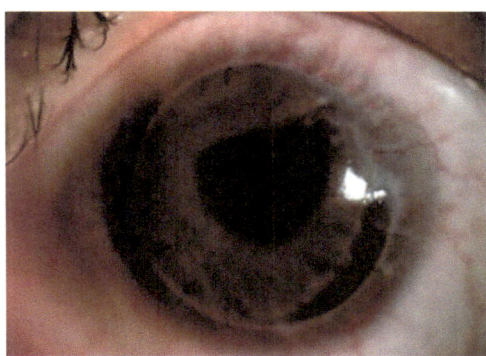

2. *Penetrating keratoplasty*: Penetrating keratoplasty is the first choice for patients
   in late stage with infection involved in the whole layers of the corneal stroma
   (Figs. 7.9 and 7.10).

After the surgery, the patients should be followed up closely, and the therapy of
anti-amoebic medicines is continued for at least 3 months. The eye drop of cyclosporine A 1% or tacrolimus 0.1% can be used after surgery, but glucocorticoid eye
drops generally should be not used in one month after surgery.

7.4   Typical Case Reports

7.4.1   Case 1: Bilateral *Acanthamoeba* Keratitis Related to Orthokeratology

A healthy 20-year-old male Canadian college student, who studied in Beijing city,
complained of redness, pain, and blurred vision in both eyes for half a month. The
patient wore overnight orthokeratology lens for 4 years and always rinsed his lenses

by tap water in Canada. When he came to Beijing University to study half a year ago, he still rinsed the lenses with tap water and then immersed the lenses with lens care solution as usual.

He experienced red eyes and pain in both eyes during last 2 weeks. After being diagnosed with viral keratitis and receiving treatment by topical antibiotic and antiviral eye drops in a clinic of the school hospital, the symptoms of the patient were not improved. Because of increasing eye pain and poor vision in both eyes, he was referred to the Department of Ophthalmology of Beijing Tongren Hospital on December 5, 2006. Ophthalmologic examination: The uncorrected vision was 8/20 in the right eye and 4/20 in the left eye. Mild swelling of the eyelids in both eyes was found. Severe ocular irritation was observed for both eyes, along with moderate congestion of the conjunctiva. No obvious discharge was found in the conjunctival sac. Slit lamp examination revealed *pseudodendrites* in the central area of the cornea in both eyes. *Multiple radial keratoneuritis* were present in the superficial peripheral cornea. Anterior chamber contained no aqueous flare, and diameter of the pupil was approximately 3 mm in both eyes (Fig. 7.11a, b).

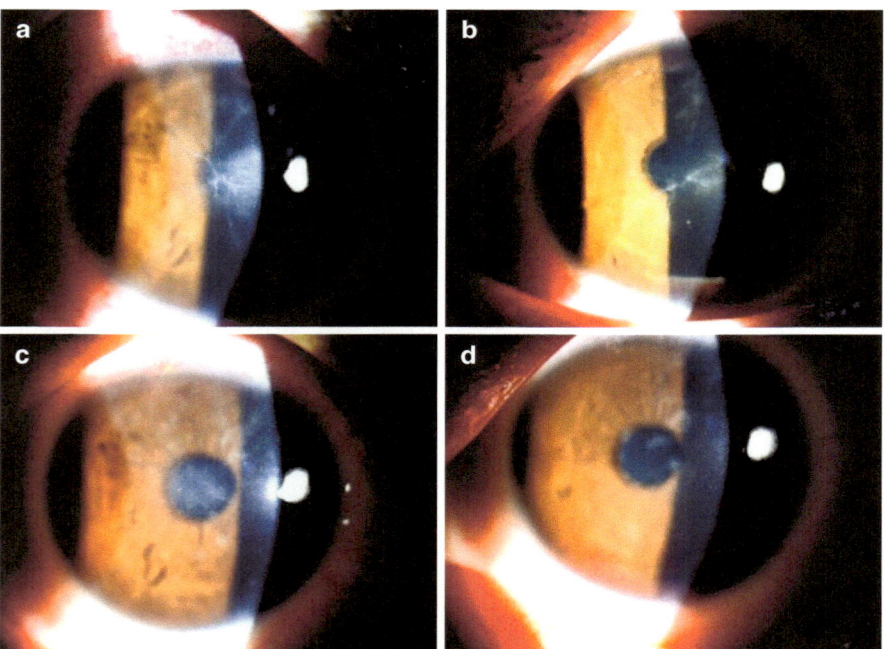

Fig. 7.11 Before treatment, pseudodendrites and radial keratoneuritis in both eyes were found (**a**: right eye; **b**: left eye). After 1 month treatment, the mild corneal nebula was formed in both eyes (**c**: right eye; **d**: left eye)

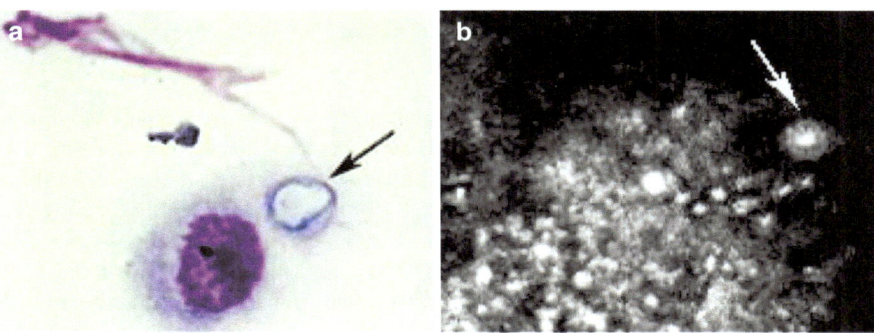

Fig. 7.12 (**a**) An *Acanthamoeba* cyst (shown by black arrow) was detected in the smear of the corneal scraping examination (Giemsa-stained, magnification ×1000). (**b**) An *Acanthamoeba* cyst (shown by white arrow) was observed in the corneal shallow stroma by the corneal laser scanning confocal microscope

Laboratory examination: A*canthamoeba* cysts can be detected in the smear examination of the corneal scraping in both eyes (Fig. 7.12a). Amoebic cultivation from the corneas in both eyes and from the lens care solution in his lens cases showed positive result. Meanwhile bacterial and fungal cultivations from the corneas in both eyes were negative. By the corneal laser scanning confocal microscope, several *Acanthamoeba* cysts were observed in the corneal shallow stroma (Fig. 7.12b).

The diagnosis was bilateral *Acanthamoeba* keratitis at early stage and the management included the debridement of the corneal lesions in both eyes and eye drops of chlorhexidine 0.04% and neomycin 0.5% once per hour for 48 h continually. After 2 weeks of treatment, the eye drops were tapered to six times per day. At noon and night, propamidine isethionate (Brolene) eye ointment 0.1% was applied.

After 1 week of treatment, the ocular irritation was significantly diminished, and the pseudodendrites in the central cornea disappeared, and multiple radial keratoneuritis was moderated. The eye drops of chlorhexidine 0.04% and neomycin 0.5% were tapered to four times per day for next 1 month. After 3 months of treatment, the corneal mild nebula was formed in both eyes, and the corrected vision acuity in both eyes was 18/20 (Fig. 7.11c, d).

Suggestions (1) Generally most of bilateral *Acanthamoeba* keratitis is related to contact lens wear, and, in trauma-related cases, bilateral infection by *Acanthamoeba* is rare. As for patients wearing orthokeratology lenses, rinsing the lenses with tap water is one of the most important risk factors. Rinsing any kind of contact lenses with tap water should be avoided. (2) For the patients at early stage, the combination of anti-amoebic medicines is the regular regimen of therapy, and debridement of the cornea lesions will help in the reduction of the amount of pathogens within the corneal tissues and penetration of medications into the corneal stroma.

7.4.2   Case 2: *Acanthamoeba* Keratitis Related to Vegetant Trauma

A healthy 39-year-old male farmer complained of redness, pain, and blurred vision in the right eye for half a month. He was accidentally struck in his right eye by corn leaf segment during farm work half a month ago. At that time, he immediately wiped the eye with a wet towel and did not experienced the discomfort in the right eye. However, he had eye redness 3 days later and consulted a physician in a clinic. Chloramphenicol eye drop 0.5% was applied three times a day. After 1 week of therapy, the symptom was not improved. Because of increasing eye redness, pain, and blurred vision, he was referred to an ophthalmologist in a local city hospital. Then he received topical antibiotic eye drops for suspected bacterial keratitis.

With progressively severe symptoms and ulceration of the right cornea, he was referred to us. The vision acuity was 2/200 in the right eye and 10/20 in the left eye, respectively. Slit lamp examination revealed diffusive congestion of the conjunctiva and the central corneal ulcer of 3 mm in diameter without hypopyon in the anterior chamber (Fig. 7.13a). Intraocular pressure was 12 mmHg in the right eye and 14 mmHg in the left eye. The smear examination of the corneal scraping by Giemsa stain contained the amoebic cysts, and the corneal confocal microscope revealed the amoebic cyst structures. *Acanthamoeba* keratitis in the right eye (at early stage) was diagnosed. The patient received topical PHMB 0.02% and chlorhexidine 0.02% w once per hour for 48 h (in day and night). After 2 weeks of treatment, both of the eye drops were tapered at 2-hour intervals during the day, and gatifloxacin eye gel 0.3% was added at night. Tropicamide phenylephrine ophthalmic solution was applied for mydriasis twice a day.

After the next 3 weeks of therapy, the corneal ulcer was healed, and the edema of the corneal stroma disappeared. (Fig. 7.13b. Both the eye drops of anti-amoebic drugs were tapered to six times per day. During the next 1 month of therapy, PHMB 0.02% was discontinued when cysts in corneal stroma were not observed by the corneal laser confocal microscope, and chlorhexidine 0.02% was administered three times per day combined with fluorometholone eye drop 0.1% two times per day until the corneal nebula was formed. The uncorrected visual acuity was 5/20 for the right eye.

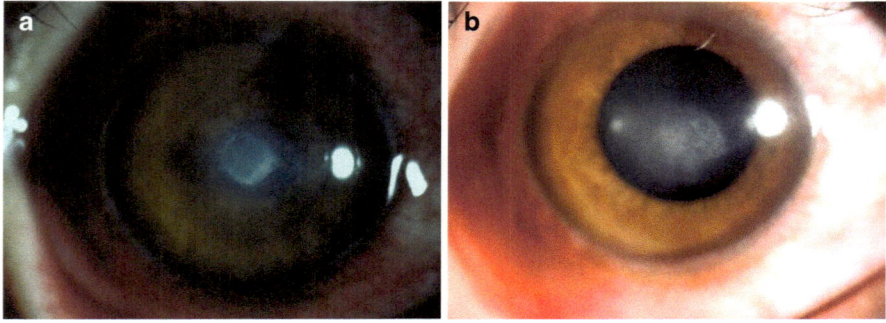

Fig. 7.13   (**a**) The corneal ulcer of patient with *Acanthamoeba* keratitis before treatment. (**b**) The corneal nebula was formed after treatment

Suggestions (1) At early stage, *Acanthamoeba* keratitis is often misdiagnosed as bacterial or viral keratitis, and generally antibiotics or antiviral medicines cannot control the amoeba infection. (2) Anti-amoebic eye drops should be used once per hour at initial treatment and tapered gradually according to the efficacy of the treatment. (3) Unless and until no cyst in the corneal tissues is observed by the corneal confocal microscope, doctors should be very careful in applying topical glucocorticoids during treatment.

7.4.3 Case 3: *Acanthamoeba* Keratitis Coinfected with Fungal Infection

A 59-year-old male surgeon in a university hospital complained about photophobia, eye pain, and decreasing vision acuity in the right eye for 2 months. He had not a history of the keratitis. He was accidentally struck in the right eye by the splash of gypsum debris 2 months ago when he was sawing the gypsum used for a fractured left leg of a patient. He experienced immediately pain in the right eye and received antibiotic eye drop for 1 day with no further symptoms. After 3 days, he had eye redness and increasing pain and blurred vision and consulted an ophthalmologist in the local eye hospital. Because of suspicion of bacterial keratitis, he received the multidrug therapy of antibiotics. However, patient intolerance required termination of this therapy after 2 weeks without benefit.

Because fungal hyphae were observed from the smear examination of the corneal scraping, he was diagnosed with fungal keratitis and received therapy with eye drops of antifungal drugs (natamycin and fluconazole). During the following 1 month of therapy with antifungal drugs, the indolent ulcer and inflammation did not resolve, with negative culture of bacteria and normal intraocular pressure. He was referred to Beijing Tongren Hospital. The vision acuity was 2/200 in the right eye and 20/20 in the left eye, respectively. The conjunctiva of his right eye showed diffuse conjunctival injection. Slit lamp examination revealed the corneal ulcer to be 7 mm in diameter with grayish-white suppuration in the central deep stroma and diffuse infiltration in the peripheral cornea. Anterior chamber contained numerous cells and a small hypopyon (Fig. 7.14a), and tactile tension was normal in the right eye. No abnormality was observed in his left eye.

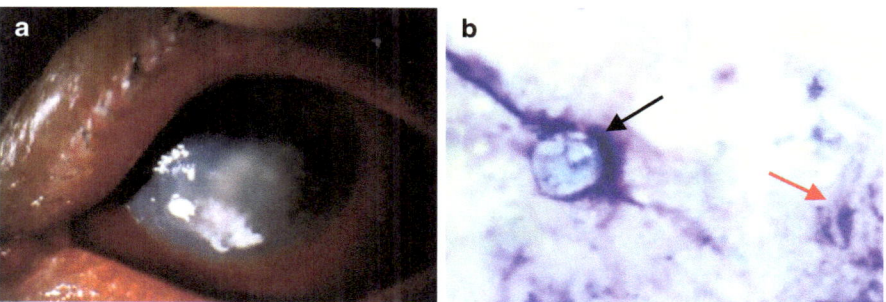

Fig. 7.14 (**a**) Corneal ulcer with the stromal infiltration in the patient of *Acanthamoeba* keratitis coinfected with fungus before the treatment. (**b**) *Acanthamoeba* cyst (shown by black arrow) and fungal hypha (shown by red arrow) were observed in the corneal smear (Giemsa-stained, ×1000)

The Giemsa-stained smears of the corneal scrapings contained fungal hyphae and *Acanthamoeba* thick-walled cyst, approximately 10 μm in diameter (Fig. 7.14b). But cultivations for fungi and amoebas were negative. No other microorganisms were detected. *Acanthamoeba* keratitis coinfected with fungus in the right eye was diagnosed based on the positive examination of the corneal smear, and the patient was admitted to the Beijing Tongren Hospital.

Eye drops of chlorhexidine 0.02% and natamycin 5% and ketoconazole 0.1% were initiated four times per day, respectively, for five consecutive weeks, with oral itraconazole (200 mg/day) for 2 weeks. Meanwhile, atropine eye ointment 1% was given for mydriasis once a day. The cautery of the corneal ulcer with iodine 5% was applied in the right eye for two times per week for two consecutive weeks. Repeat smear of the corneal scraping did not contain fungi hyphae and amoeba cysts after 5 weeks of therapy; subsequently eye drops of anti-amoebic medicines were gradually tapered from six times a day to two times a day. During the next 3 months of therapy, the corneal ulcer was healed, the inflammation of the corneal stroma disappeared gradually, and the corneal nebula was formed in the right eye.

Suggestion (1) *Acanthamoeba* keratitis coinfected with other microorganisms is not common. Both *Acanthamoeba* keratitis and fungal keratitis have similar risk factors, process of onset, and clinical manifestations, differential diagnosis alone based on the clinical manifestations is relatively difficult. The correct diagnosis mainly depends on laboratory microbiological examination. Especially the repetition of the corneal smears can help detect coinfected pathogens and adjust the therapeutic regimen during the treatment. (2) Antifungal drugs and amoebicides should be applied simultaneously for patients with coinfection of fungus and amoeba. As for the cases with indolent corneal ulcer and severe inflammation in anterior chamber (numerous cells and hypopyon), an oral antifungal drug should be given. (3) Because *Acanthamoeba* cysts may remain in the corneal tissues for a long time, the total duration of therapy should be at least 6 months with gradually tapering of anti-amoebic eye drops, in order to avoid relapse of infection.

7.4.4   Case 4: *Acanthamoeba* Keratitis Caused by a Splashed Insect

A healthy 28-year-old male farmer complained of redness and pain with blurred vision in the left eye for 2 months. A small flying insect splashed into the left eye of the patient when he worked in the farm fields. After wiping the eye with a wet towel, he only experienced a mild foreign body sensation and did not go to visit his physician. After 1 week, because of the redness and grinding sensation with blurred vision and severe pain in his left eye, he presented to a local hospital. With him being diagnosed with suspected bacterial keratitis, he received the therapy of multi-antibiotic eye drops. After 3 weeks of therapy with antibiotics, because of progressively severe symptoms and indolent corneal ulcer, he was transferred to a city

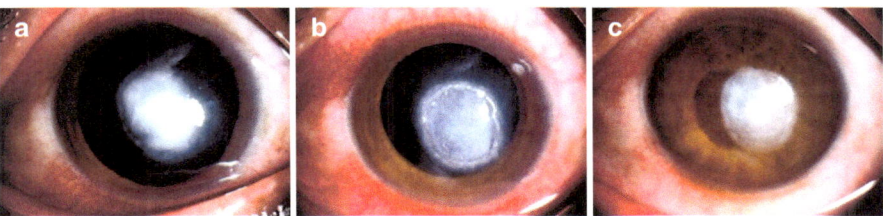

Fig. 7.15 (**a**) The corneal ulcer of patient with *Acanthamoeba* keratitis before treatment. (**b**) After the lamella excision of the corneal lesion. (**c**) The corneal macula was formed one and a half month after surgery

hospital and was diagnosed with fungal keratitis based on the fungal hypha in the smear examination of the corneal scraping. After treatment for 2 weeks with eye drop of natamycin 5%, the corneal ulcer was protracted. He was referred to us. The vision acuity was 20/20 in the right eye and 2/200 in the left eye. The diameter of the central corneal ulcer was about 5 mm with dense infiltration in the deep corneal stroma, but the peripheral cornea was clear (Fig. 7.15a). No hypopyon in anterior chamber was observed. The intraocular pressure was 16 mmHg in the right eye and 20 mmHg in the left eye. The right eye was normal.

Acanthamoeba cysts were observed in the smear examination of the corneal scraping, and the cultivation of amoeba from the corneal scraping yielded *Acanthamoeba* without other microorganisms. With diagnosis of *Acanthamoeba* keratitis in the left eye at advanced stage, the therapy with eye drops of chlorhexidine 0.02% and neomycin 0.5% was given as described above. After therapy with anti-amoebic drugs for 2 weeks, the lamella excision of the corneal lesion was carried out in order to reduce the amount of pathogens and improve the healing of the corneal ulcer (Fig. 7.15b). After the lamella excision of the corneal lesion, eye drops of anti-amoebic medicines were continued and gradually tapered to three times per day. When the patient was followed up after one and a half month of therapy, the corneal macula was formed with clear anterior chamber (Fig. 7.15c). With discontinuation of instillation of neomycin 0.5%, the eye drop of chlorhexidine 0.02% was continually used twice a day for the following 3 months.

Suggestions (1) Shallow lamella excision of the corneal lesion cannot only remove the necrotic tissues of the corneal ulceration but also eliminate the pathogens or reduce the amount of pathogens in the corneal tissues. The antigen of pathogens in the corneal tissues could induce immune reactions and aggravate the inflammation. Therefore, the shallow lamella excision of the corneal lesion can also help in reducing infiltration and repairing the corneal tissues. (2) During the lamella excision of the corneal lesion, one should be careful with the depth of excision in order to avoid the perforation of the cornea. (3) After the surgery, the application of amoebicide eye drops generally is required for at least three following months. Meanwhile, antibiotic eye drop should be added for prophylaxis of bacterial infection.

7.4.5   Case 5: *Acanthamoeba* Keratitis Related to Orthokeratology

A healthy 27-year-old female graduate student consulted to Beijing Tongren Hospital with complaints of redness and pain in the left eye, accompanied by decreasing vision acuity for 1 month. She had history of orthokeratology (night wear) lens wear for more than 10 years and did not clean the lenses regularly in recent years. One month ago, she visited a local hospital due to redness and grinding sensation in the left eye and was diagnosed with viral keratitis. With the therapy of antiviral and antibiotic eye drops for 2 weeks, the condition of the disease was aggravated, and tobramycin and dexamethasone ointment was added once at night. After 1 week, she was referred to us. The visual acuity was 10/20 in the right eye and hand movement in the left eye. Slit lamp examination revealed the ulcer of the center area of the deep corneal stroma to be 5 mm in diameter, with diffused congestion of the conjunctiva in the left eye. A small hypopyon in anterior chamber was observed and tactile tension was normal (Fig. 7.16a). *Acanthamoeba* cysts were detected in smear cytologic examination of the corneal scraping and through corneal laser confocal microscopy of the left eye.

Acanthamoeba keratitis in the left eye was diagnosed, and the eye drops of chlorhexidine 0.04% and polyhexamethylene biguanide (PHMB) 0.04% were given once per hour, respectively. After 3 weeks of treatment, the indolent corneal ulcer did not resolve, and the patient had increasing eye pain. Therefore, surgical treatment was required. Corneal transplantation was carried out 3 days later. The culture of amoeba from corneal fragments was positive. After the surgery, chlorhexidine eye drops 0.02% was applied for six times per day for 3 weeks and gradually tapered later. After 1 month of surgery, fluorometholone eye drop 0.1% was added three times a day for 2 weeks and then discontinued. The topical prednisolone phosphate 1% was given three times per day. In the follow-up of 10 months after surgery, the corneal graft was clear (Fig. 7.16b), and the uncorrected visual acuity in the left eye was 15/20.

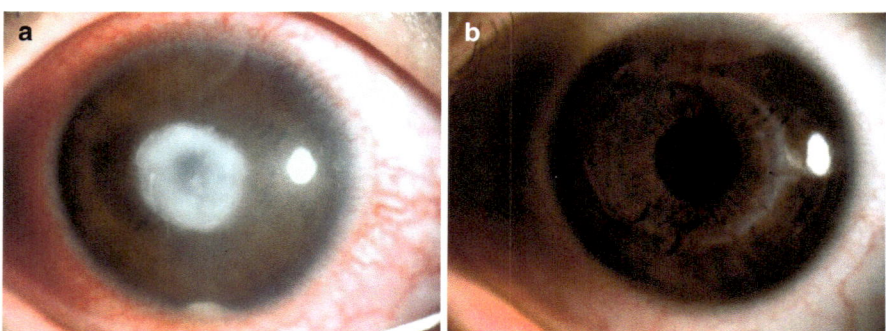

Fig. 7.16 (**a**) The corneal ulcer of *Acanthamoeba* keratitis with mild hypopyon before surgery. (**b**) The transparent corneal graft after 10 months of surgery

Suggestion (1) Pathogenic amoebic protozoa have been detected in tap water. Therefore, it is recommended that rinsing with tap water should be avoided for all types of corneal contact lenses in order to reduce the rate of the amoebic infection. (2) If patients at advanced stage have no improvement with the therapy of anti-amoebic drugs after 4 weeks of treatment, surgical treatment should be considered. If patients progress to the late stage, the corneal transplantation should be recommended immediately. (3) After surgery, the eye drops of amoebicides should be continued at least for 3 months, combined with eye drops of cyclosporine A 1% or tacrolimus 0.1%. Topical corticosteroid should be avoided in 1 month of surgery.

7.5   Dispensing Method of Anti-amoebic Eye Drops in Hospital

Chlorhexidine Eye Drops
Bulk pharmaceutical chemicals: chlorhexidine gluconate 20%
    Solvent: glucose solution 5%
    Concentration of eye drops: 0.02%, 0.04%
    Dispensing method:

1. Chlorhexidine eye drop 0.02%: 0.5 ml of chlorhexidine gluconate stock solution 20% is taken and added to 500 ml of glucose solution 5%. These two ingredients are mixed evenly and sub-packaged in sterile ophthalmic bottles that are kept in the condition of avoiding light.
2. Chlorhexidine eye drop 0.04%: 1 ml of chlorhexidine gluconate stock solution 20% is taken and added to 500 ml glucose solution 5%. These two ingredients are mixed evenly and sub-packaged in sterile ophthalmic bottles that are kept in the condition of avoiding light.

Neomycin Eye Drop
Bulk pharmaceutical chemicals: neomycin sulfate powder
    Solvent: sterilized saline solution
    Concentration of eye drop: 0.5%
    Dispensing method:
    Five mg of neomycin sulfate powder is added to 100 ml saline solution. Once the powder is completely dissolved, the solution is sub-packaged in sterile ophthalmic bottles that are preserved at room temperature.

PHMB Eye Drops

Bulk pharmaceutical chemicals: PHMB stock solution 20%
    Chemical name: polyhexamethylene biguanide hydrochloride
    Solvent: glucose solution 5%
    Concentration of eye drops: 0.02%, 0.04%
    Dispensing method:

1. PHMB eye drop 0.02%: 0.5 ml PHMB stock solution is taken and added
   to 500 ml glucose solution 5%, which are mixed evenly. The mixed solution is sub-packaged in sterile ophthalmic bottles and kept in the condition
   of avoiding light.
2. PHMB eye drop 0.04%: 1 ml PHMB stock solution is taken and added to
   500 ml glucose solution 5%, which are mixed evenly. The mixed solution
   is sub-packaged in sterile ophthalmic bottles and kept in the condition of
   avoiding light.

Metronidazole Eye Drop

Bulk pharmaceutical chemicals: metronidazole disodium phosphate for injection (powder injection).
    Solvent: sterilized saline solution or glucose solution 5%.
    Concentration of eye drop: 2%
    Dispensing method:
    0.915 g metronidazole powder injection (actually containing 0.862 g met-
ronidazole) is added to 43 ml sterilized saline solution or glucose solution 5%
and mixed evenly. These ingredients are sub-packaged in sterile ophthalmic
bottles and are preserved at room temperature.

It is recommended that the eye drops should be prepared before use. The storage
period of prepared eye drops is generally 2 weeks. The preparation and dispensing
process should be performed in a relatively sterile environment, such as operating
room or sanitized outpatient treatment room. Chlorhexidine and PHMB eye drops
have to be kept in the condition of avoiding light. The clarity of the eye drops should
be checked before instillation. If there are precipetations observed in the eye drops,
the patients should immediately stop application.

References

1. Perrine D, Chenu JP, Georges P, et al. Amoebicidal efficiencies of various diamidines against
   two strains of *Acanthamoeba polyphaga*. Antimicrob Agents Chemother. 1995;39(2):339–42.
2. Brasseur G, Favennec L, Perrine D, et al. Successful treatment of *Acanthamoeba* keratitis by
   hexamidine. Cornea. 1994;13(5):459–62.

3. Byers TJ, Kim BG, King LE, et al. Molecular aspects of the cell cycle and encystment of *Acanthamoeba*. Rev Infect Dis. 1991;13(Suppl 5):S373–84.

4. Ogbunude PO, Asiri SA. In vitro effect of diamidines on intracellular polyamines of *Acanthamoeba polyphaga*. Drugs Exp Clin Res. 2001;27(4):127–33.

5. Johns KJ, Head WS, O'Day DM. Corneal toxicity of propamidine. Arch Ophthalmol. 1988;106(1):68–9.

6. Larkin DF, Kilvington S, Dart JK. Treatment of *Acanthamoeba* keratitis with polyhexamethylene biguanide. Ophthalmology. 1992;99(2):185–91.

7. Lee JE, Oum BS, Choi HY, et al. Cysticidal effect on *Acanthamoeba* and toxicity on human keratocytes by polyhexamethylene biguanide and chlorhexidine. Cornea. 2007;26(6):736–41.

8. Elder MJ, Kilvington S, Dart JK. A clinicopathologic study of in vitro sensitivity testing and *Acanthamoeba* keratitis. Invest Ophthalmol Vis Sci. 1994;35(3):1059–64.

9. Xuguang S, Yanchuang L, Feng Z, et al. Pharmacokinetics of chlorhexidine gluconate 0.02% in the rabbit cornea. J Ocul Pharmacol Ther. 2006;22(4):227–30.

10. Mathers W. Use of higher medication concentrations in the treatment of *Acanthamoeba* keratitis. Arch Ophthalmol. 2006;124(6):923.

11. Seal DV, Hay J, Kirkness CM. Chlorhexidine or polyhexamethylene biguanide for *Acanthamoeba* keratitis. Lancet. 1995;345(8942):136.

12. Guzek JP, Roosenberg JM, Gano DL, et al. The effect of vehicle on corneal penetration of triturated ketoconazole and itraconazole. Ophthalmic Surg Lasers. 1998;29(11):926–9.

13. Savani DV, Perfect JR, Cobo LM, et al. Penetration of new azole compounds into the eye and efficacy in experimental Candida endophthalmitis. Antimicrob Agents Chemother. 1987;31(1):6–10.

14. Osato MS, Robinson NM, Wilhelmus KR, et al. In vitro evaluation of antimicrobial compounds for cysticidal activity against Acanthamoeba. Rev Infect Dis. 1991;13(Suppl 5):S431–5.

15. Casemore DP. Sensitivity of Hartmannella (Acanthamoeba) to 5-fluorocytosine, hydroxystilbamidine, and other substances. J Clin Pathol. 1970;23(8):649–52.

16. Varga JH, Wolf TC, Jensen HG, et al. Combined treatment of *Acanthamoeba* keratitis with propamidine, neomycin, and polyhexamethylene biguanide. Am J Ophthalmol. 1993;115(4):466–70.

17. Khunkitti W, Lloyd D, Furr JR, et al. *Acanthamoeba castellanii*: growth, encystment, excystment and biocide susceptibility. J Infect. 1998;36(1):43–8.

18. Hay J, Kirkness CM, Seal DV, et al. Drug resistance and *Acanthamoeba* keratitis: the quest for alternative antiprotozoal chemotherapy. Eye (Lond). 1994;8(Pt5):555–63.

19. Duguid IG, Dart JK, Morlet N, et al. Outcome of *Acanthamoeba* keratitis treated with polyhexamethyl biguanide and propamidine. Ophthalmology. 1997;104(10):1587–92.

20. Radford CF, Lehmann OJ, Dart JK. *Acanthamoeba* keratitis: multicentre survey in England 1992-6. National *Acanthamoeba* Keratitis Study Group. Br J Ophthalmol. 1998;82(12):1387–92.

21. Hargrave SL, McCulley JP, Husseini Z, Brolene Study Group. Results of a trial of combined propamidine isethionate and neomycin therapy for *Acanthamoeba* keratitis. Ophthalmology. 1999;106(5):952–7.

22. Xiuying J, Luo S, Yang B, et al. Investigations on the diagnosis and treatment of *Acanthamoeba* keratitis. Chin Ophthalmic Res. 2000;18(2):143–5.

23. Sun X, Zhang Y, Li R, et al. *Acanthamoeba* keratitis: clinical characteristics and management. Ophthalmology. 2006;113(3):412–6.

24. Xuguang S, Xiuying J. *Acanthamoeba* keratitis. Ophthalmol CHN. 2002;11(1):4–6.

25. McClellan K, Howard K, Niederkorn JY, et al. Effect of steroids on *Acanthamoeba* cysts and trophozoites. Invest Ophthalmol Vis Sci. 2001;42(12):2885–93.

26. Seal DV. *Acanthamoeba* keratitis update-incidence, molecular epidemiology and new drugs for treatment. Eye (Lond). 2003;17(8):893–905.

27. John T, Lin J, Sahm D, et al. Effects of corticosteroids in experimental *Acanthamoeba* keratitis. Rev Infect Dis. 1991;13(Suppl 5):S440–2.

28. Park DH, Palay DA, Daya SM, et al. The role of corticosteroids in the management of *Acanthamoeba* keratitis. Cornea. 1997;16(3):277–83.

29. Illingworth CD, Cook SD, Karabatsas CH, et al. *Acanthamoeba* keratitis: risk factors and outcome. Br J Ophthalmol. 1995;79(12):1078–82.

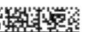

30. Lee GA, Gray TB, Dart JK, et al. *Acanthamoeba* sclerokeratitis: treatment with systemic immunosuppression. Ophthalmology. 2002;109(6):1178–82.
31. Wang H, Qu G. Research advance of Miltefosine. Cent South Pharm. 2006;4(6):454–6.
32. Walochnik J, Duchene M, Seifert K. Cytotoxic activities of alkyphosphocholines against clinical isolates of *Acanthamoeba* spp. Antimicrob Agents Chemother. 2002;46(30):695–701.
33. Kishore P, Gupta S, Srivastava DK, et al. Action of methylglyoxal bis (guanyl hydrazone) and related antiprotozoals on *Acanthamoeba culbertsoni*. Indian J Exp Biol. 1990;28(12):1174–9.
34. Gatti S, Cevini C, Bruno A, et al. In vitro effectiveness of povidone-iodine on *Acanthamoeba* isolates from human cornea. Antimicrob Agents Chemother. 1998;42(9):2232–4.
35. Jiang J, Yao K, Zhang Z. Evaluation on the toxic effect of different concentration of povidone iodine to rabbit cornea (domestic products). Chin J Ophthalmol. 2006;42(4):338–40.
36. Hughes R, Dart J, Kilvington S. Activity of the amidoamine myristamidopropyl dimethylamine against keratitis pathogens. J Antimicrob Chemother. 2003;51(6):1415–8.
37. Codling CE, Maillard JY, Russell AD. Aspects of the antimicrobial mechanisms of action of a polyquaternium and an amidoamine. J Antimicrob Chemother. 2003;51(5):1153–8.
38. Kilvington S, Hughes R, Byas J, et al. Activities of therapeutic agents and myristamidopropyl dimethylamine against Acanthamoeba isolates. Antimicrob Agents Chemother. 2002;46(6):2007–9.
39. Chen H, Liu W. Clinical application of novel antifungal medicine caspofungin Foreign Medical Sciences Section of Dermatology and Venereology. 2005;31(1):9–11.
40. Bouyer S, Imbert C, Daniault G, et al. Effect of caspofungin on trophozoites and cysts of three species of Acanthamoeba. J Antimicrob Chemother. 2007;59(1):122–4.
41. Guo Y, Wang J, Zhengtang C. Recent advancement in pharmacological effects of artemisinin and its derivatives. Chin J Clin Pharmacol Therap. 2006;11(6):615–20.
42. Nacapunchai D, Phadungkul K, Kaewcharus S. In vitro effect of artesunate against *Acanthamoeba* spp. Southeast Asian J Trop Med Public Health. 2002;33(Suppl 3):S49–52.